Helping Your Overweight Child

Helping Your Overweight Child

A FAMILY GUIDE

Caroline J. Cederquist, M.D.

Advance Medical Press

Library of Congress Control Number: 2001-133124

ISBN: 0-9714164-0-0
Cover Design: Pearl & Associates
Book Production: Tabby House
Printed in the United States of America

Author's Note

The information provided in this book is based on my experience and should not replace the advice of your health-care provider. It is not the intent of this book to diagnose or prescribe treatment but to help you assist your child to become healthier and to manage weight problems, in cooperation with your child's personal physician. The dietary recommendations in this book can be followed by all children, not just those who are overweight. Only your personal physician can determine if this nutritional lifestyle plan is suitable for your child. Take your child for periodic checkups and professional supervision. Address to your child's health-care provider any questions or symptoms that may arise.

Please understand that should you use the information and recommendations contained in this book without your doctor's approval, you are prescribing for yourself, and the publisher and the author assume no responsibility.

CAROLINE J. CEDERQUIST, M.D.

Publishers Cataloging in Publication
(Provided by Quality Books)

Cederquist, Caroline J.
    Helping your overweight child : a family guide /
Caroline J. Cederquist. -- 1st ed.
    p. cm.
    includes bibliographical information and index.
    LCCN 2001133124
    ISBN 0-9714164-0-0

    1. Obesity in children. 2. Children--Nutrition.
3. Eating disorders in children. I. Title

RJ399.C6C44 2002   618.92'398
                                    QB101-701250

Advance Medical Press
853 Vanderbilt Beach Road #342
Naples, FL 34108

Dedication

To Ed, Melissa, and Jessica, thank you for all your loving support.

Acknowledgments

First, without the invaluable editorial labors of Carole J. Greene, this book would not exist. I also called upon friends to read early versions of the manuscript and would here like to thank Dick Bruno and Rhona Saunders for their wise counsel and insightful suggestions. Primarily, I want to pay tribute to my patients, from whom I learned more than I could possibly attribute in this or any other published work.

I owe a debt of gratitude to the faculty members of Fairfax (Virginia) Family Practice Center, where I initially learned all about family practice. These skilled, caring professionals embraced me in the kind of nurturing environment I had only dreamed I would find in my career. My thanks also go to the American Society of Bariatric Physicians, which has been instrumental in fostering my focus and education in the field of weight management.

Throughout my life, my parents—Catherine and Neale Szabo—always encouraged my academic endeavors and provided a loving safety net that allowed me to soar without fear of landing hard. They knew I was ready to tackle this book even before I did.

Foreword

Childhood and adolescent obesity is an ever-increasing problem that has multiple long term societal and individual consequences. In more than twenty years of family practice I have seen far too many attempts to deal with obesity fail, despite the best of intentions. Weight-control programs are too often focused on short-term fixes and very few focus on the problems that are specific to this age group. As a parent of teens, I have witnessed the challenges our children face as they form the habits that shape their lives. Dr. Cederquist's book is a welcome and refreshing answer to these concerns.

It is a sensible book—the approach to diet and exercise is not about fads or short-term gains—it is about establishing lifelong habits that will help your child and your family. The suggestions relate to choices about day-to-day things—not regimens of foods and activities that are hard to maintain.

It is a personal book—the stories and examples are easy to relate to and illustrate the very personal factors that influence the myriad of individual decisions that build healthy habits.

It is a family book—this more than anything else makes this book stand out. Family involvement is the essential ingredient that is missing from so many other approaches. Dr. Cederquist's recommendations are good for supporting healthy habits, and are good for families in general.

This book has the essential ingredients for long-term success: identification of predictable challenges, easy-to-follow recommendations for diet and exercise, and practical suggestions for family involvement. It is a book that will work for your child and your family.

CRAIG CLARK, M.D.

Contents

Chapter Three: K.C. and Her Family Take "Nutrition 101"

Chapter Four: K.C. Tackles Exercise

Chapter Five: K.C. Bugs Her Family to Change

Chapter Six: K.C. Faces a Crisis

Chapter Seven: K.C. Reaches Her Goals

Appendix One

Appendix Two

Appendix Three

Appendix Four

Appendix Five

Index

One

K.C. Has a Problem

Kelly stumbled into the house, her eyes red and swollen. She slammed the door shut and rushed to her room. She switched on the computer to see what was happening in her favorite Internet chat room. Soon, she knew, her mother would be framed in the doorway of her bedroom. The door slam would have alerted her that Kelly had a problem.

While the computer booted up, she threw herself onto her bed and reached for the economy size bag of peanut M&Ms on her bedside table. Her full mouth would give her a few seconds to think how to respond to her mother's accusation about the door slam. She wouldn't compound her problems by talking with her mouth full.

"Kelly," her mother began, "you know better than to slam the door. What's with you?"

"Don't call me Kelly!" the girl said once her mouth was empty. "I hate my name!"

Her mother approached the bed. "Why, Kelly Camille Wilkes, you can't be serious. For eleven years you've always loved your name."

"Well, I hate it now. Find something else to call me. My initials or something."

Her mother sat beside her on the bed. "I don't understand, Kel—I mean, K.C. What's going on?"

"Oh, Mother," K.C. began. She looked down at her hands, as if for the first time noticing the bag of candy. Tears slid down both cheeks.

"Go on, sweetheart, what is it?" The mother put her arm around K.C.'s

1

shoulder and pulled her close. "Whatever it is, let's face it together."

K.C. took a deep breath. "All the way home from school—on the bus—those terrible boys who live down the street from us made fun of me. Billy and Johnny."

"Yes. What did they say?"

"They didn't *say* anything. They sang it. A song they made up. About me." Again, K.C.'s eyes filled and overflowed.

Her mother patted her leg. "You know that 'Sticks and stones may break your bones but words will never hurt you.' So what could they say—sing—that would be so terrible?"

K.C. sat up straight, as if trying to fill herself with courage. She took a deep breath. "They kept singing, over and over, 'Kelly the belly, so round and fat. See the Grand Canyon? That's where she sat!' That's why I hate my name. Why couldn't you name me something that doesn't rhyme with anything? Especially anything that means I'm fat!"

Mrs. Wilkes sat quietly for a moment. "Oh, honey, I'll call you K.C. if that will make you happy. But it's not your name that you hate, it's your weight. We talked about this a few weeks ago, remember? How you have the same shape as Grandma Wilkes."

"Yeah, I know. I've seen her pictures lots of time. And she was always as big as the Metlife blimp."

Mrs. Wilkes grimaced. "Yes, I'm afraid so. Well, dear, when you take after someone like that, you know you need to watch what you eat—like those M&Ms on the table there."

K.C. nodded, her sobs subsiding. "I know, but . . . ."

"No buts, you're just going to have to go on a diet."

"Not another stupid diet, Mother. That will just make the kids tease me more. Please, no."

"This time, I won't put you on a diet I cut out of a magazine. I'll make an appointment with the doctor and ask her to help us."

"The last diet didn't help. I'm still fat. How can the doctor help?"

"I don't know, but let's find out."

* * *

This little story demonstrates what typically happens to get a patient into my office to confront a weight problem. The child didn't become heavy overnight. Rather, the weight gain sneaked up on her. It required a slow process, a complex interaction of genetic, behavioral, and environmental factors. But it often takes a wake-up call before the child and her family are ready to face the situation.

Sometimes it's cruel taunts from a child's acquaintances. Or maybe a parent's concern that her child is too heavy. The wake-up call could be a visit from a relative who hasn't seen the child for a couple of years, whose eyes widen at the child's size. Even a trip to the swimsuit department in the spring could trigger the awareness of a weight problem. No matter what the reason, I see in my family practice more and more overweight youngsters.

And no wonder. Since 1970 the number of overweight children in the United States has more than doubled![1] Now, approximately one in five children in this country between the ages of six and seventeen is overweight.[2] North of our border, statistics published in the August 26, 2000, edition of the *Windsor Star* indicate that obesity among Canadian children aged seven to twelve soared in the 1990s. Obesity in that age range rose to 23 percent from the former figure of 15 percent.[3] According to a recent article in *Pediatric Alert*, this disturbing trend toward obesity has to be among the most serious of the major problems facing pediatrics in the early 21st century![4]

All these statistics become even more meaningful in light of our culture's preoccupation with twig-thin models!

Throughout this book, we'll be talking about our fictional "Kelly"—okay, we'll do as she asked and call her "K.C."—and her family. We could just as easily have chosen "Kevin" to represent the heavy child who will provide the focus of our weight-management efforts. The statistics tell us that the figures for child and adolescent obesity are about equally distributed between boys and girls. However, because the emotional burden of being overweight falls more heavily on girls, we'll follow K.C. as she moves through the course of this book from overweight and emotionally miserable to normal in weight and happy in attitude. When we use the feminine pronouns, replace them with the masculine ones if the child you are helping is a boy. As you read the vignettes that demonstrate what's going on with K.C., substitute your child's name. This will help you make the emotional investment necessary to help your child.

We know you want to help your child. Caring about your child's weight problem moved you to pick up this book, just as the concern the health-care professionals in my office have for our patients—and the millions of children like them—compelled us to write it. My staff, including nutritionists and exercise physiologists, and I will "talk" to you in this book the way we would if you were in our office. Together, we *will* make a difference.

Let's get started!

What Has Caused the Rise in Childhood Weight Problems?

According to statistics compiled from various sources, 27 percent of the children in this country, and 21 percent of adolescents, would be classified as "obese." This represents a 54 percent and a 39 percent increase, respectively, since 1970. As just noted, the childhood obesity rate is similar in Canada, making it a North American cultural problem.

Because "obese" and "obesity," medically correct words, carry negative emotional feelings for most people in this culture, we will limit our usage of them as much as possible. However, it is important for you to know what health-care professionals mean when they use "the O words."

Obesity Defined

Obesity is a chronic, debilitating, and potentially fatal disease marked by an excess accumulation of body fat in a quantity sufficient to endanger health. (As we shall see, a variety of factors determines what is meant by "excess" fat.) Recognized since 1985 as a chronic disease, obesity is the second leading cause of preventable death, exceeded only by cigarette smoking.[5] The excess accumulation of body fat results from an imbalance between energy intake and energy expenditure. In other words, we put on weight, in the form of stored fat, when we eat more calories than we use up in our daily activities.

The treatment of obesity has spawned a whole branch of medical specialization called bariatric medicine. As a board certified bariatric physician, as well as a family physician, I devote a large segment of my private practice to weight management and to the patients, like your child, who need a compassionate partner in their struggle to manage their weight.

What has made K.C.—and your child—heavier than nature intended? Let's look at the story that opened this chapter. Our vignette demonstrates the three primary factors that produce more energy intake than energy output: 1) poor food choices; 2) inactivity; and 3) problems in home, school, or social environments. In the vignette, K.C. suffers emotional stress from taunts about her weight—an environmental factor. As a "comfort food," K.C. reaches for a large bag of M&Ms. Not the best food choice. Because "chatting" on the Internet is one of her favorite pastimes, we can assume that she doesn't get much exercise. In this scene from K.C.'s life, she's batting a thousand! A negative thousand, that is.

In order to return her weight to the level that nature intended for her, our K.C.—and yours—will need to make some adjustments in her life.

How Do I Know What My Child's Weight Should Be?

Before you undertake wholesale changes in the way your family lives, you will want to know if your child is truly "overweight." If K.C.'s body shape looks like that of "Grandma Wilkes," she may always be on the large side. Or maybe she's about to shoot up in an adolescent growth spurt, which will normalize her weight in relation to her height. To find out if significant lifestyle changes are necessary—or maybe even medical intervention—take your child to your family physician or pediatrician.

You probably remember the old height-weight charts that divided the population into male and female, and then small, medium, or large boned. Today's weight charts don't talk about the size of bones, as we'll see in a minute.

Overweight children usually don't bother with bone size either. They're much more inclined to see themselves as just plain fat. In reality, our bodies are made up of various kinds of tissue. In addition to our bones—no matter what size!—we have organs (heart, stomach, intestines, etc.), muscle (sometimes referred to as lean body mass), blood and other fluids, and—yes—fat.

You see, fat itself is not a bad thing. In ancient times, fat often meant the difference between life and death for our forebears. When hunting and gathering were successful, our distant ancestors ate the plentiful food and stored up fat in their bodies to carry them through the months when snow and cold made gathering impossible and hunting difficult. That's the way our bodies are designed—to store fat in good times for survival in lean ones.

However, today's sophisticated society no longer relies on the body's ability to store fat for usage when food isn't plentiful. There's always more at a nearby grocery store! Too bad that our bodies haven't changed since ancient times, so that we still store as fat the energy we don't need at the moment.

So your doctor won't use the old height-weight charts to determine whether your child's body is storing too much energy as fat. Instead, your health-care professional will measure your child's height and weight and, using a set formula, calculate the BMI, or body mass index.

This BMI has become the accepted way of measuring health risk related to excess weight. Why? Because it provides a useful tracking history of weight relative to height. As children in weight-management programs grow taller, we want to see the BMI numbers come down, not necessarily their weight.

Just introduced to physicians are revised growth charts, including two new body mass index-for-age charts—one for boys and another for girls—ages two to twenty. (See charts on pages 6 and 7.) Physicians use these charts to measure the presence of obesity, both in individuals and in the general population. The American Society of Bariatric Physicians (ASBP) tells us that the charts will also be utilized in studies to establish national overweight prevalence estimates and to monitor progress toward achieving the country's national "Healthy People" goals for the year 2010.[6]

Likewise, our northern neighbors will use statistics gathered from the use of such charts to draw attention to the obesity issue. Obesity Canada, a nonprofit group composed of health professionals, notes that the federal and provincial governments are just now beginning to realize the impact of lifestyle issues such as obesity. This organization understands that the disturbing trend toward obesity and its resultant health problems could add billions of dollars to the annual cost of the country's Medicare system.[7]

Most professionals will use these charts as an educational tool to help parents understand their child's growth patterns. The BMI-for-age charts explain patterns of adequate or inadequate growth, identify goals for change, and evaluate and reinforce changes in growth over time. Expect your health-care professional to remind you that the general growth pattern over a period of time is more important than a single measurement plotted at any one visit to the office.

BMI Charts

These are the charts that physicians use to determine whether a child's weight is appropriate for her/his height.

Definitions: overweight = BMI at 95th percentile; at risk for overweight = BMI at 85th percentile but under 95th. This may seem confusing to you, but your healthcare professional will know how to use this index.

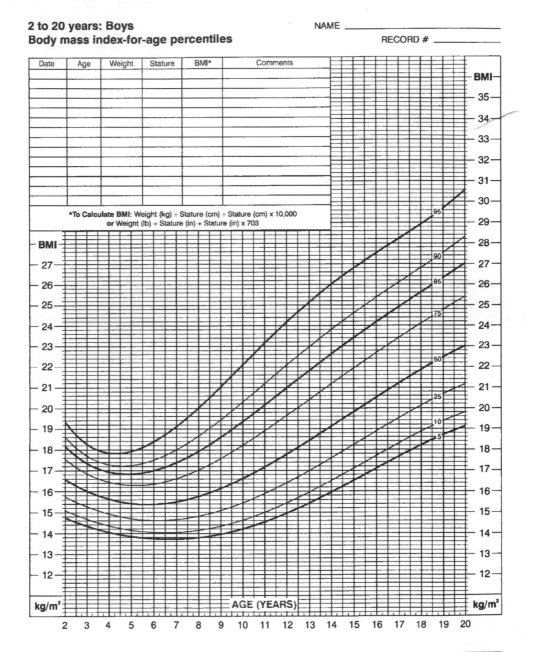

SOURCE: Developed by the National Center for Health Statistics in collaboration with
the National Center for Chronic Disease Prevention and Health Promotion (2000).
http://www.cdc.gov/growthcharts

In older children and adolescents, the BMI has a close relationship to body fat. Because of this, the index indicates high or low levels of fat mass. This indicator is significant to determine those persons who, *at an early age*, might benefit from weight management programs.

After determining your K.C.'s BMI, the doctor will ask several questions related to how she lives, eats, exercises, whether there are any stressful situations in the fam-

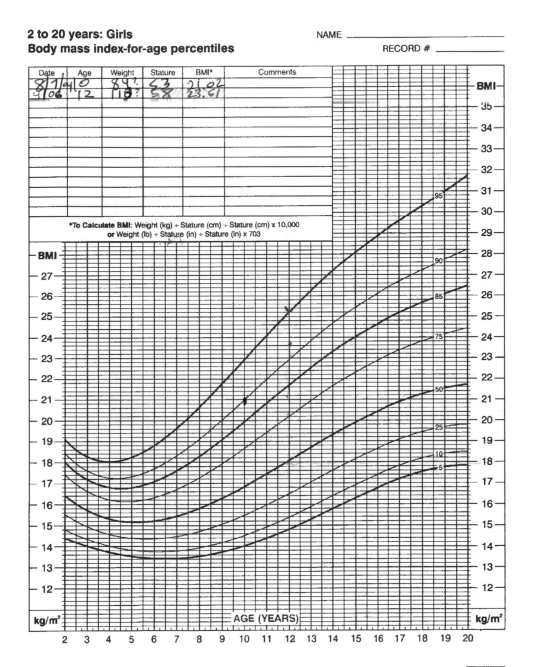

2 to 20 years: Girls
Body mass index-for-age percentiles

NAME _____

RECORD # _____

*To Calculate BMI: Weight (kg) ÷ Stature (cm) ÷ Stature (cm) x 10,000
or Weight (lb) ÷ Stature (in) ÷ Stature (in) x 703

ily, and your family's emotional attitudes toward weight. Don't be surprised if you are asked about the health of your marriage, as an impending divorce, or the stresses of single parenthood, for example, can cause your child to overeat. (More about this later in the book!) Be prepared to talk about Grandma Wilkes and other relatives who always carried excess pounds. Yes, genetic inheritance plays a significant role.

Biology and Genetics

Even if your K.C. takes after the heavy side of the family, that realization does not have to carry with it a burden of guilt. In fact, knowing that "it's not *all* my fault" can help children in their struggle against overweight!

Lately, science has discovered that just as genetics determines your child's hair color and texture, eye color and vision acuity, genetic make-up *does* significantly affect whether your child will be inclined to be overweight, normal or thin.

How do we know this? Researchers have studied the body weights of adults who were adopted as infants and reared by adoptive parents. They compared the body weights of these adults with the weights of both their biologic parents and their adoptive parents. The adoptees' weight and body types were more similar to those of their biologic parents than to those of their adoptive parents. [9] Studies of identical twins who were reared apart show more similarities than differences with regard to weight and body type.

What Do We Inherit That Relates to Our Weight?

So what do we inherit from our forebears? First is the tendency to store energy as fat. This comes from the interaction of many of the body elements that determine how much energy we burn while at rest, which is called **metabolism**.

This was nicely demonstrated in several studies where investigators compared the resting energy expenditure—metabolism—of infants and young children of overweight parents to the metabolism of children with normal weight parents. An equal number of infants and children in both groups were normal weight, overweight, or thin. However, the researchers found that the children of overweight parents had a lower metabolism than did the children of non-overweight parents. [10]

Another study found that normal weight four-year-old children of overweight parents had a lower intake of calories, a lower rate of calories burned during exercise, and lower metabolic rates than did normal weight four-year-olds born to normal weight parents.[11] To put it bluntly, it's just as you've always suspected: children of overweight parents need fewer calories to maintain their weight. If they eat the same amount of food as their friends who have thin parents and thin genes, they gain weight.

When your K.C. complains, "Sara can eat everything and still she's a stick, but if I walk past a doughnut shop, I gain a pound," she's not far off!

Also inherited are components of your appetite and your satiety—the feeling of fullness you have after you have eaten. Some adults and children feel hungrier than others and need more food to reach that feeling of satisfaction. However, some appe-tite and satiety factors are learned. How? Possibly from well-meaning parents who encourage their kids to clean their plates. Or from long-standing family traditions coupled with tasty foods—for example, the weekly dinner with the grandparents that presents four kinds of homemade pasta topped off with delicious pastries. It is also true that some children with insatiable appetites eat for emotional nourishment rather than out of actual hunger. We'll go into greater depth about this subject later in the book.

You also inherit where on the body to store excess fat. Think of your extended family. Can you identify any pattern that repeats through several generations—such as thin arms and legs but excess fat on the abdomen or heavier thighs and hips? Do the grandchildren show the same fat-storage characteristics as Grandma? Genetics! You knew it!

The general literature shows that if one parent is overweight, half of the children in the family will be overweight. If both parents are overweight, approximately two-thirds of their children will be obese.

Don't you just hate statements like that? They don't bode well for your kids if you parents have passed along these genes. Such information can, however, alleviate some of your guilt and pain. You—and your children—are not entirely to blame.

However, you're not completely off the hook for guilt and anger over genetic tendencies. If your overweight child's body shape and size make him look like Great Uncle Charlie—whom you never could stand—you may have to work extra hard not to let it bother you that your child reminds you of this relative. Acknowledge your emotions so that your child won't bear the brunt of these negative feelings. Parents of overweight children need to exercise caution in the comments they make so that they don't inadvertently blame the children for their hereditary tendencies. Let them know that people come in lots of different shapes and sizes, all of them natural.

If your children have the biological susceptibility to gain fat easily, they may never be "thin." It will be up to you, the parents, to help your children accept the body type they have, even though it does not meet the current cultural ideal.

Okay, so, because of genetics, your kids will never be stick-thin. But **neither are they doomed to struggle with their weight for the rest of their lives!** In order for that to happen, the genetic susceptibility must be coupled with an environment that promotes weight gain. You play an important part here, too, as you help to create that environment. Throughout this book you'll learn much more about creating a healthful family environment.

Family Composition

Let's look at a few other results of studies on obesity. It has been found that over-weight is more common in *only* children or *firstborn* children. Overweight is much less prevalent in larger families than in smaller families. Children living with a single parent have also been found to have a higher rate of overweight than do children from a family with two parents. Children born to parents who are older than the norm for childbearing have an increased likelihood of overweight problems.[12]

The reasons for the above correlations are not clear cut. All probably have a multitude of contributing factors. What is clear is that attitudes and behaviors about food and exercise are present in every family. Some families develop very positive eating behaviors while other families develop more negative ones that increase the likelihood of weight problems.

Determining whether your child's weight results strictly from heredity that is not in your control or from environmental factors that can be altered is *not* easy! That's why we urge you to consult a physician, who can help sort out the various factors that need to be addressed as you help your K.C.

How Dangerous Is It If My Child Is Overweight?

Aside from the emotional upheaval and poor self-esteem your K.C. must endure from the cruel taunts of her acquaintances, what difference does it make if she's overweight? A *huge* difference in her medical well-being!

Obesity has been established as a major risk factor in the occurrence of such diseases as diabetes, hypertension (high blood pressure), cardiovascular disease (heart and circulatory system), and some cancers, particularly of the breast and colon. Diabetes itself can lead to life-threatening and debilitating complications such as blindness, end-stage kidney disease, nerve damage, limb amputation, heart attack, and stroke. Obesity may produce apnea, a frightening condition in which the person temporarily stops breathing while asleep. Excess weight puts more burden on the skeletal system, resulting in joint problems, such as arthritis and dislocations of the hip.

Do you want your child to grow into the kind of adult who would suffer from such conditions? Of course not.

In the Bogalusa Heart Study, researchers looked at the relationship between cardiovascular risk factors and overweight in children ages five to seventeen. They found that overweight children had a higher incidence of elevations in their cholesterol, blood pressure, and fasting insulin. The study concluded that "because overweight is associated with various risk factors even among young children, it is possible that the successful prevention and treatment of obesity in childhood could reduce the adult incidence of cardiovascular disease."[13]

Your K.C., should her weight problem continue, could be at risk for one or more of these chronic diseases. But add to that the emotional factors, and the problem looms even larger. The psychological consequences of a child's being overweight are just as serious as the medical ones. From as early as kindergarten, children develop negative views of their overweight classmates. Often, children describe overweight people as lazy, stupid, or slow. Couple this with our culture's media bombardment of unreasonably thin supermodels to represent the ideal of beauty, and it's no wonder that we see youngsters becoming depressed—even suicidal—because they're too heavy. They start to hate themselves, which turns into failure at school, failure to make friends, failure to care about what happens to themselves or their families. Disaster may not be far away.

You can be glad about whatever triggered you to pick up this book. Together, we can keep these dire predictions from coming true for your child!

Let's Get Started by Defining Goals

1. *No "Diets"*

The very first goal I'd like to suggest is that you *not* talk about putting your K.C. on a diet. We are ALL on a diet, because the original definition of that word is: what we eat! With our society's preoccupation with thinness, we have started to think that the only meaning of the word *diet* is a regulated, restrictive list of allowable foods intended to drop pounds. No wonder K.C. hates the idea of being on a *diet*! We all hate it.

Rather, I'd like you to think in terms of **healthy food choices**, as opposed to poor food choices. And healthy activities, as opposed to sedentary ones, positive emotional attitudes instead of negative ones. Helping your family develop nutritious eating patterns they can follow throughout life is far more important than following a weight-loss regimen.

Also, as we proceed to suggest changes in your K.C.'s behaviors, our treatment goal will be to slow down the rate of her weight gain. Weight loss may not be recommended for children, unless they are significantly overweight. Instead, we will focus on weight maintenance, or slowing down how fast weight is gained.

Most children, especially girls, gain body fat as they approach puberty. Often, this extra fat is lost when the child reaches her next growth spurt. Although this change in height and weight may continue over several years, it most frequently occurs within an eighteen- to twenty-four-month span. During this rapid growth period, your child needs increased nutrients—a good reason *not* to be on a restrictive weight-loss type of diet. If you concentrate on maintaining your child's weight during this time, when she hits that growth spurt she should have adequate fat stores to allow growth into a normal weight as her height increases.

So don't think "diet." Instead, think "maintain until the growth spurt."

2. *Get In Touch With Your Feelings*

Look back to the first words of this chapter, at the vignette that introduced K.C. and her mother. Did you get the idea that Mrs. Wilkes wasn't fond of her mother-in-law? That she thought of her negatively because she believed her to be the progenitor of K.C.'s weight problem? Do you think K.C. would have liked or disliked her grandmother, had she known her? How much might her mother's attitude toward her grandmother influence K.C.'s feelings?

Do *you* have any negative feelings toward someone in your family who has a weight problem? If you do, don't fret. Just honestly admit that you have these feelings.

Maybe not out loud and in public, but to yourself. "I guess I've never gotten along with Aunt Maude because I thought she was lazy and slow, when really all she is fat. I might feel better about her if I saw her as unable to conquer a complex problem that involves heredity and environment, instead of lacking willpower or desire."

Once you acknowledge your feelings toward this overweight relative, the next goal is to be aware of how you feel about your overweight child. Does some of that same negativity fall onto her? Do you perhaps focus on all the bad things your child does and maybe not see all the good? This can happen if you feel strongly that your child should be closer to today's ideal of beauty—thin to the point of emaciation.

If your self-examination indicates you have had negative feelings toward your child because she is heavy, don't beat yourself up, commit yourself to change. **Tell your child that she is okay, no matter what she weighs. Say it out loud and often.**

How children feel about themselves often depends on how their parents feel about them. So let your child know that your love is unconditional. Point out all her good qualities—her lovely smile, her enthusiastic laugh, the neat way she keeps her room, her talent at the piano—whatever is true of *your* child.

Let your K.C. know that children come in many shapes and sizes, and none of them is inherently *wrong*. **Your child is more important than what she weighs!** Show her respect, love, attention. Hug her. Talk with her. Comfort her with love, not with food. Praise her for specific reasons and tell her what they are. Every day!

3. *Develop Your Child's Self-esteem*

All of this will go a long way toward the next goal: Help your child develop self-esteem. When you demonstrate positive feelings toward your child, she will notice and will take them into consideration when looking at her own feelings about herself.

Talk with your child about her weight and encourage her to share her feelings on the subject whenever they arise. Feelings are not to be ignored. When your child opens up to you, realize that she is taking a risk of rejection. Listen to her. Really focus all your attention on what she's saying, instead of glancing at the TV or puttering around the kitchen while she's sharing her innermost fears or hopes. Reassure her that no matter what pain or frustrations she feels and expresses, she is still okay, still lovable.

Throughout the remainder of this book, we will detail changes that your K.C. and the entire family will commit to making in order to reach and maintain the weight that nature intended for her. Making a commitment to change requires self-esteem. If a child doesn't care about herself, she can't muster the courage and persistence to produce change.

We do not expect you to become a psychologist and examine every behavior to assess whether it fosters self-esteem. As we go along, we'll help you understand what positive behaviors to establish and what negative ones to abolish.

4. *Write It Down*

We have found in our treatment of overweight patients that one of the most helpful tools is to keep a journal. Until you've done it, you have no idea how therapeutic it is to put down on paper your feelings—hopes, desires, fears, frustrations. This doesn't have to become a dreaded chore. Instead, it can be simple jottings.

If your K.C. is of an age where she can read and write, ask her to keep her own journal. If your child is too young, then you keep it for her. She can note her feelings at various times of the day and what she did about them. For example, in our vignette, K.C. came home crying from being teased by the neighbor boys. How did she react? She reached for the M&Ms!

When your child starts keeping a journal, she will be able to see how and when food might be used to fill an emotional void. Emotions occupy a large part of the intricate tapestry that makes up obesity. Once your child starts to see the patterns, she can begin to make appropriate substitutions for the comforting food.

Take a few moments now to turn to the appendix. Look at our suggested format for your child's journal. Note that it contains three elements: eating, exercise, emotions. Your K.C. will establish and work toward goals in each of those areas, just as our patients do when they come to our office. We know this process of setting goals has worked for them. It can work just as well for you and your K.C.

Chapter Recap

* If your child is overweight, she is not alone. She is but one of the 4.5 million overweight youngsters in the United States aged six to seventeen—>20 percent of the population in that age range. Statistics for Canadian youngsters are similar.

* The leading causes of overweight in children are: poor food choices, inactivity, and problems in their environment coupled with genetic susceptibility.

* If you are concerned about the weight of your child, consult with your health-care professional, who will calculate your child's BMI to determine whether your child has a weight problem that needs to be addressed. (See appendix to learn how to calculate your own or your child's BMI.)

* Genetics plays an important role in our body shape and size, our tendency to store energy as fat, our metabolism, and our appetite and satiety levels. Realizing that "it's not their fault" helps many children to deal more positively with being larger than their peers.

* Being overweight has been shown to lead to other chronic diseases, such as diabetes, high blood pressure, heart disease, and some cancers. Psychological and emotional problems can be just as devastating to the medically overweight person as any of these chronic diseases. However, if addressed during childhood, obesity does not have to become a lifelong struggle.

* *Initial Goals: Don't think "diet"; Get in touch with feelings—your child's and your own; Help your child develop self-esteem; Show your child how to keep a journal.*

Two

K.C. Learns What Made Her Fat

K.C.'s father stood at the foot of the stairs and called, "Come on, K.C., or we'll be late for the movie."

"Okay, Daddy. Be right down." She put a clip in her hair, her favorite—the one her father said he liked. She felt good today. Her dad, home from his week on the road, was taking her and two of her friends to a movie. And for this weekly "date with Dad," she didn't have to take along her little brother Kyle. She wouldn't have to put up with Kyle's relentless teasing about her weight. But even better, she would have her father's full attention. It would be a very good day.

Before her daughter could come downstairs, Mrs. Wilkes took her husband aside. "Honey, it's not too late to go skating instead. Kelly really needs to get some exercise. All she does during the week is study, watch TV, and go on the computer. I'd like her to have some activity."

"Oh, please, Ellie. I'm tired. I had a hard week. Then yesterday I spent hours playing catch with Kyle. Can't I have a little relaxation with my daughter just one day a week?"

Ellie shrugged. "I suppose so. But I know the two of you at the movies. Promise me you'll try to watch what she eats today, okay?"

"Yeah, yeah. Hey—here's my girl now. Bye, honey. Bye, Kyle. Let's go Kel—uh—K.C."

At the Cineplex, K.C. stood in line at the refreshment counter, gabbing and giggling with her friends Sara and Alexa. When they got to the head of the line, she caught her father's eye. "Go ahead. Get the jumbo popcorn," her dad said, "with lots of butter the way you and I like it. You get free refills with the jumbo size, and I know the way you three girls can sock it away. And four Cokes."

"I want a Diet Coke," Sara said.

"Me, too," Alexa copied.

K.C. slid a twenty to the freckle-faced clerk. "Jumbo with loads of butter, two diets, two regulars. Make them jumbo, too."

It was a good thing, K.C. thought later, that the flick dragged in a couple of spots. It gave her time to return for a popcorn refill without missing any of the action. Only K.C. and her dad gobbled up the refill; Sara and Alexa shook their heads each time the bucket was passed to them.

Outside the Cineplex, Mr. Wilkes glanced at his watch. "Hey, pretty ladies, what do you say we slide by McDonald's for a quick supper. Or are your parents expecting you home?"

"That's okay, Mr. Wilkes," Sara said, "I'm not hungry. That popcorn filled me up."

"Me, too," said Alexa, "and my folks want me home for supper? My grandmother's coming over."

K.C. looked grim. She was having such a good time with her father, she didn't want it to end. "Tell you what, Dad, let's drop Sara and Alexa at their homes and you and I go to McDonald's."

Mr. Wilkes threw his arm around his daughter's shoulders. "Sounds great. You know how much I look forward to spending time with you on the weekends. So it'll be just the two of us." He put up his hand for a high five.

K.C. slapped his hand with her own. "Yeah, no Kyle to bug us."

Over their supersized Big Mac meals, Mr. Wilkes reviewed his week on the road. K.C. laughed at his humorous tales of sales appointments, computer glitches, and order screw-ups. Her dad, jolly and talkative, was good at customer relations. When his office sometimes made mistakes, he was always able to patch things up with his customers. "I take 'em out for lunch and after a couple of beers, they're in a much better mood," he explained, patting his own considerable beer belly.

He mopped his mouth with a napkin. "Had enough? I think I'll go for a hot fudge sundae. How about you?"

K.C. paused for a moment. She felt full, but she wouldn't see her daddy for five more days. Eating together like this was a joy for her. For him, too. "Sure, Dad, get one for me."

When they got home, Mrs. Wilkes and Kyle were clearing the supper dishes. "I'll bet you two had a great time," her mother said.

Kyle stuck his tongue out at his big sister. She glared him into submission. "Yeah," K.C. reported. "The movie was super; I had a real good cry at the sappy ending. Then we dropped off the girls and went to McDonald's."

Mrs. Wilkes sighed. "What did you order? I'll bet you five dollars you supersized it, whatever it was."

"Now, Ellie, don't get on her case. If you want to blame anyone, blame me."

"I do blame you. Look at the two of you. If you're not two peas in a pod, I don't know what is. It isn't bad enough that she inherited your stocky build, you have to encourage her to overeat—and undo all the trouble I go to during the week to get her to eat healthy."

"Ellie, I . . ."

"Don't 'Ellie' me. You have as much of a weight problem as she does, even if you do carry it well. Didn't the doctor tell *you* to lose fifty pounds? You shouldn't be eating at McDonald's. Not unless you choose the salad. Did you? Did you get the salad?" One look told her the answer. "I thought so. I don't mind your eating at a fast-food place—I certainly take the kids there during the week when you're gone—but you both know you're supposed to make the healthiest choice available. We've been over and over this."

Bill Wilkes tried not to look sheepish. "You're right. I didn't think. We were having such a good time, I didn't want to spoil it by demanding that we 'eat healthy'."

Ellie Wilkes shook her head. "You make 'eating healthy' sound like a prison sentence. I thought we were all agreed, that this was a family decision to help K.C. with her weight problem—and you."

"Yeah, but the Big Mac and fries taste so much better."

"I do not intend to give up on this. Do you want her to wind up like your mother? Suffering all those years with diabetes and heart trouble. Then dying at forty-eight?"

Her husband shook his head. "No, of course I don't."

"K.C. does just fine during the week when you're not here. She's learning how to make better food choices. Then you come home and in one day turn everything upside down. You're supposed to be the adult, the mature one who helps solve problems. Instead, you're doing just the opposite."

"Look, Ellie, I don't want to fight about it. You're right. I'm wrong. Let's just leave it at that. I promise to do better."

Ellie looked at her daughter, who had stayed so quiet they forgot she was there. "Hear that, K.C.? No more Big Mac meals, super sized or not."

"Yes, Mother, I hear."

* * *

Poor K.C.—caught between a mother concerned about her weight and a father who, overweight himself, continues to follow his poor eating habits. Our vignette develops several themes here:

* Most kids usually go along with whatever is suggested by the dominant person in a crowd.
* Children and adolescents have a need to be liked and accepted greater than the need to always watch their diet.
* Alexa and Sara know when they've had enough—they aren't dealing with the same emotions K.C. has, nor with the same metabolism or satiety levels.
* If it's tough for adults—supposedly more mature and responsible—to give up a Big Mac and fries in favor of a healthier choice, then how hard must it be for a child!

Typical Childhood Eating Situations

We have purposely created a family that demonstrates many of the situations we encounter in our office. In today's fast-paced life, one parent (in this case, the father) is so busy with earning a living that he leaves nearly all the family situations to the mother. K.C. does have a strong bond with her mother and wants to follow her food guidelines, but when Daddy is home on weekends, they both become "junk food junkies." Loving to eat is about the only thing they have in common. They share the same inherited slower metabolism, the same higher satiety level, so they're both overweight.

Even Mrs. Wilkes succumbs to the ease and convenience of relying on fast food. When she's had a hard day, it's much easier to take the family to a restaurant than to go to the trouble of preparing a meal at home.

Our Fast-Food, Fast-Life Culture

This, too, is representative of our current culture. Over the past twenty years, the dietary habits of our culture have changed considerably. These changes directly contribute to the rise in obesity! Statistics show that three-quarters of all meals are eaten outside the home.[1] In 1997, meals and snacks taken away from home captured 45 percent of the U.S. food dollar, up from 39 percent in 1980 and 34 percent in 1970. [2]

Why should it make a difference in our weight that more meals are eaten outside the home? First, restaurants offer larger portion sizes than we eat at home, probably to justify their prices. Second, in order to make the foods taste better—so we'll return again and again—restaurant chefs use greater amounts of sodium, sugar, and fat than we probably would at home. Another element is the "bargain" deal that is hard to pass up. When we can "super size" our soda and fries for a few pennies more, why not! After spending considerable time at restaurants, some families unconsciously increase their portion sizes when eating at home, to make those servings more consistent with the restaurant meals.

Most people, by nature, are "completers." If we are given a larger portion, we finish it. After all, it is right there in front of us and paid for. Or, like the jumbo popcorn and soda at the movies, refills are free.

Changes In Our Family Dynamics

The last twenty years have also seen a change in family dynamics. Many, if not most, families now require both parents to work in order to provide a comfortable standard of living. That results in less time available to prepare homemade foods and increases reliance on restaurants and prepackaged foods. It is not unusual for parents to get home late, and one or all of the children need to attend some event in the evening. What happens? The family cannot eat together, so they resort to grabbing a "fend for yourself" meal. This often takes the form of processed foods higher in sugar and fat, like a peanut butter and jelly sandwich with a bowl of ice cream. Maybe in your house it's a ham and cheese sandwich with chips and dip. Or a frozen meal that can be zapped in the microwave. Such quickie meals *can* be planned to pay attention to nutrient content, but most tend to be higher in fat and lower in fiber than recommended. Check the appendix for a list of our "better" picks.

Celebrations—Fast Foods and Virtual Games

In our vignette, K.C. and her father go to McDonald's. We could have used any other fast-food restaurant, and the message would be the same: this is a place we like to go when we feel happy and want to celebrate being together. In fact, lots of places now capitalize on this "celebrate with us" concept. In many towns the local movie palace has a party room, where you can arrange a birthday party for your child and several friends. Not only will it include a movie, but also as much junk food as the little tikes can hold. A new crop of arcades has blossomed, offering computerized and video "virtual" games that the kids adore, plus, of course, the party room along with the low nutrient food. In these places, they've never heard of carrots and celery, only high-fat foods and high-sugar drinks.

Is it any wonder that our K.C.—and yours—easily gets to be twenty or thirty pounds overweight?

Too Much Intake, Too Little Output

So far, we've concentrated on the eating, or intake, end of the quotient. Now let's look at the other end— the output. Remember, we noted in chapter 1 that obesity results from taking in more energy than you use up, with the excess energy stored as fat. Our K.C., and millions like her, exercises too little to expend the energy she consumes. She loves to read, watch TV, or sit at her computer for hours—remember the chat room we mentioned in the first vignette? Millions of other children do the same. When K.C. and her father went out together, they saw a movie. They could have gone skating instead, as the mother suggested. But they didn't.

Millions of other families make the same kinds of choices—sedentary over active—video games at an arcade that *show* action instead of sports that require us to *be* active. It's part of the culture and hard to deny. This topic is important enough to deserve its own chapter—chapter 4.

Parental Attitudes Regarding Weight

K.C. is caught between a mother overly concerned and watchful of every bite she puts into her mouth and a father whose eating habits have contributed to his own weight problem. K.C. is not dangerously overweight, and her father hates to be too restrictive with her during the rare moments they spend together. He doesn't object that she is learning to make healthier choices—he understands that this kind of lifestyle change will benefit her forever. Also, he figures that she is likely to have a growth spurt soon and "grow into" her weight as she gains height. However, with her mother, the issue is more emotional: her mother would like K.C. to be closer to the ideal we see everywhere in our culture—the thinner the better.

"You can't be too rich or too thin." This adage represents the hallmark of current North American culture. However, thinness as a sign of wealth (demonstrating that the slender person has plenty of time to work out, perhaps with a personal trainer, or visit such pricey indulgences as health spas) is a fairly recent phenomenon. A couple of hundred years ago, when the plump Rubenesque figure was in vogue, carrying excess weight was a sign of affluence. The common people were too poor to have much to eat. Only the people in the aristocracy could afford to eat well enough to develop a paunch!

Times have changed. Today, our ideal of beauty—celebrities, movie and TV stars, and fashion models—sometimes look thin to the extreme, even emaciated. With the media bombardment we are subjected to, is it any wonder that we crave thinness for ourselves and for our loved ones?

In fact, because the ideal of beauty in today's society requires protruding bones without even an ounce of meat on them, we have seen an appalling rise in eating disorders. The prevailing attitude, especially among adolescent girls, is "Thin at any cost," even when the cost results in bulimia and anorexia! We will detail eating disorders, their signs and what to do if you suspect your child may be heading for one, in chapter 6.

Often, well-meaning parents can play a role in pressuring a child to lose weight. They may emphasize the pain and ridicule an overweight child must endure to the extent that their child resorts to behavior that develops into an eating disorder.

That's why, when a family comes to our office with concerns about the weight of a child, we ask questions to ascertain how the parents feel about their child's weight. We counsel our parents not to place their own fears and ideals of body shape and weight onto their children. Consequently, we also look for warning signs that the child may be involved in the kind of activities that signal an eating disorder.

Parents need to be aware of their children's habits and personalities. If either changes—say, your child becomes depressed or moody when she used to have a happy disposition—she may be headed for trouble. Youngsters most prone to eating disorders tend to be perfectionists, who want to control every aspect of their lives. We'll cover this subject more fully in chapter 6.

Making Healthier Choices

Most children should not follow restrictive weight-reduction diets unless their weight puts their overall health in jeopardy. They should focus on learning to make healthier choices and allow their next growth spurt to even out their weight/height values.

What do we mean when we advise our patients to make healthier choices? In our office, we suggest to our patients and their families several specific changes that really are not difficult but can make a big difference in eating habits.

Change Takes Time

Remember that change occurs slowly. Don't expect to alter a lifetime of eating habits in a few days. It will take weeks or months before new patterns and behaviors become routine. But our K.C. and yours did not put on excess weight overnight, so we won't demand that she become what nature intended her to be in just a few brief weeks.

Here's the first change I'd like to recommend. Draw the family together once a week and look at the calendar for the upcoming seven days. What evenings will work, school, and other activities allow the family to eat at home together? Mark it down and ask everyone to commit to being there.

Make Mealtime Pleasant

On those nights, *make dinner a relaxing, happy event*. Switch off the TV, computer, and video games and gather around the kitchen or dining room table. Use this opportunity to get better acquainted with what's going on in everyone's lives.

Promise that no one will nag or complain. Never let mealtime—what should be a pleasant family event—erupt into scenes and arguments. If mealtimes produce stress, children tend to eat fast and leave the table as quickly as possible. Then they associate eating with stress, which leads to emotional overeating.

S-l-o-w d-o-w-n. *Make meals last more than 15 minutes*. No matter what after-dinner activities beckon, keep this a relaxing time. If everyone is talking about meaningful happenings in their lives, laughing and enjoying one another, the tendency to relax and eat more slowly will come naturally. When we eat slowly, our stomachs signal our brains that we are full before we eat more than our bodies need.

Many of our patients come to us having no idea that eating too fast makes them eat too much. It's true. Studies indicate that overweight children tend to eat twice as fast as thinner ones. To experience that feeling of satiety, we require a certain amount of tasting, sucking, chewing, swallowing. Gobbling food down as fast as possible doesn't give the brain enough time to signal "satiety level has been reached." Eating more slowly allows us to be satisfied with less food.

How to Make Mealtimes Last Longer

How can you make the mealtime last long enough to reach the satisfaction level before you eat too much? Here are some hints.

* Put your fork down between bites. Pick it up again only after you have finished chewing and swallowed. When eating finger food, such as a sandwich, put it down while you chew. Doing this automatically adds several minutes to the time it takes to finish a meal. You can do this even when eating alone.

* Chew your food completely and swallow it before you take the next bite. Ask a question of one of your companions before you take that bite, or answer a question someone has asked you.

* Once or twice during the meal, stop eating altogether for a couple of minutes. Tell a joke. Laugh. This will help break the rhythm of eating so that your stomach can signal that it's full before you overeat.

* Eat your meal in courses, beginning with the lowest calorie foods, such as salads, vegetables, or fruits. Then dine on the higher energy foods—bread, pasta, and meat. Dining in courses helps stop the urgent hunger feelings before you gobble down the foods that make you put on weight.

* If you think you want a second helping, wait five minutes before taking it. The desire may disappear. But if you do take another helping, make it *half* the size of the first one.

These are suggestions that have worked with some of our patients some of the time. We recommend that you not force any of these techniques on your family. Instead, present the reasons for eating more slowly, then suggest these as options and let them choose what to try. Some families in our weight programs have reported that the kids got higher grades because they chose to use dinner time to ask questions related to what they were studying in school! Just think of the possibilities: a healthier body *and* higher academic achievement. What a revolution!

Meal Presentation

Dining together without the TV drawing our attention may be enough of a revolution, but we're going to take it a step further. We suggest that *meals be allowed in only one or two places in the home—the kitchen or the dining room.* Try to make the table as pretty as possible, with colorful place mats and napkins, perhaps a floral arrangement in the center—either fresh flowers or artificial, as your budget allows. Depending on their ages, your kids might even make the colorful place mats, painting plain plastic ones with poster paints. Let them be creative, to make the table *their* special place.

In order not to encourage second helpings, we suggest that you *serve food from the stove*, not from bowls on the table. Having that big bowl of mashed potatoes conveniently within reach can be oh so tempting. Your K.C. might change her mind about taking more food if she has to get up from the table to do it.

Make Sure You Are Hungry

Eating only when hungry may seem like an obvious thing, but we know many people who eat by the clock, not by their body's hunger: If it's noon, it must be lunchtime.

Well, maybe not. On those lazy summer holidays, for example, when the family gets up late and has breakfast at 9:30, they won't be hungry at noon. Follow the dictum: **Don't eat if you're not hungry**. Hold off eating until your body says "it's time."

Although our metabolism—the rate at which food is transformed into nutrients to run our bodies—is largely genetic, it can be influenced by when we eat. From literature in the field of obesity studies and from interviews with patients who come to us, we know that people who eat one large meal per day gain the most weight.

It makes sense when you think about it. Let's say your K.C. skips breakfast, has only a minimal lunch or none at all. When she gets home in the afternoon, she is famished and dehydrated. Running on empty, she begins eating and doesn't stop till she goes to bed. From 3:00 to 9:00 P.M., it's all just one big meal. She may take in only the 2,000 calories recommended for her age and height, but because she takes them in all at once, she gains weight.

Why? Because of what happens inside her body. Prior to that one large meal in the evening, the body has been operating in "starvation" mode, conserving energy. Her body has become very efficient at storing energy. Then, when she takes in her daily calories pretty much all at once over several hours in the evening, her body secretes greater amounts of insulin to metabolize her food. I won't go into the medical meaning of this right now. Let's just say her metabolism becomes too efficient.

We don't *want* an efficient metabolism. Rather, we want your K.C.'s body to realize that its fuel will come in small portions and regularly throughout the day so that the body will *use it as it comes and not store energy for later.*

We teach our weight-management patients to eat several smaller meals throughout the day. Even if it means getting up a little earlier, start the day with a normal breakfast. Plan a small mid-morning snack, then have a normal lunch. It's okay for your K.C. to have a mid-afternoon snack when she gets home from school. In fact, this is an excellent time to get children used to eating fruits and vegetables. (More about this later.) When your K.C. eats at regular times throughout the day, she will actually eat *less* because she will not feel so starved.

Finally, when your K.C. joins her friends at a fast-food restaurant, she doesn't have to stand out as "different" by pulling a bag of celery and carrot sticks out of her purse or backpack. We know how important it is for youngsters to fit in with their peer group. We also understand that the desire to be accepted by friends generally outweighs the need to guard against eating too much. That's why we have included in our appendix a "best" food choices list, even when dining at a fast-food restaurant. Once your K.C. commits to making healthier choices no matter where she eats, she will find it easier to select something from the list. And she will pass up most opportunities to "super size" her meal. No matter how little it costs, for her, it is *no* bargain.

Chapter Recap

* K.C. learned that a number of elements in her life contribute to her being overweight. Some come from eating too much or the wrong kinds of food. Others come from filling emotional needs, such as wanting to be liked and accepted by her father and doing what he likes to do. Still others result from her genetic inheritance; her grandmother and her father both had problems with weight; she has to change her habits to overcome her inherited metabolism and satiety levels.

* Current lifestyle habits send us to restaurants more often than ever before. Our busy families, short on time, resort to dining out frequently, to the detriment of our diets. Restaurant food tends to be higher in fat, sodium and sugar and served in large portions. We get accustomed to this and demand the same in food consumed at home. All this has contributed to the rise in obesity.

* Too much food, too little exercise for too many people. More about exercise in chapter 4.

* Even children, and particularly adolescents, can succumb to dangerous eating disorders. Be on the lookout for warning signs. If some are present in your child, discuss the possibility with your family physician or pediatrician, who can make a referral to an appropriate counselor.

* Learn how to slow down at meals and enjoy this family time. Get in touch with what everyone is doing, tell jokes or stories, maybe even do some spelling-dictionary or geography quizzes!

* Learn to eat only when hungry; don't reach for a second helping from a too-convenient bowl on the table. Instead, serve meals from the stove.

* Regardless of the metabolism your children inherited, they can help to control it by eating regularly throughout the day. Take in the day's calories at breakfast, mid-morning snack, lunch, mid-afternoon snack and dinner. They will eat less and their bodies will not become too efficient at storing energy.

* Even when dining out, learn how to make healthier choices. See the appendix for lists.

Three

K.C. and Her Family Take "Nutrition 101"

"Thank you for coming this evening," the nutritionist said as she entered the room. "I like patients new to the weight-management program to get a good start, and these one-hour seminars really can help."

"What can we learn in one hour about solving K.C.'s weight problem?" Bill Wilkes muttered to his wife.

"You'd be surprised," Ellie answered as this evening's instructor distributed some papers. "K.C. and I have come twice already and we've learned a lot. We wanted you to come with us to this one, as you happened not to be traveling this week. So hush up and learn something. It'll do you good."

"Okay, 'Mother,' I'll be quiet." He grinned at his wife then accepted the papers she passed along.

"You'll see that the top sheet I've given you is a little quiz," the nutritionist said. "This will test your knowledge of basic nutrition facts. The results will tell us what we need to emphasize this evening. So take a few minutes and answer these questions."

K.C. read the questions. *This won't be too hard,* she thought. Everyone knows this stuff. Let's see—question one: True or False, skim milk does not have as much protein or calcium as whole milk. Hm-m-m. I think that's true.

Question two: 2% milk is low-fat, 98 percent fat free with only 2 percent of the calories from fat. True or False. My answer to that one will be true. That was easy—simple math.

Question three: 80% lean ground beef has only 20 percent of calories from fat. True or False. Duhhh. True, of course. Unless it's a trick question.

Question four: What has more sugar: A Butterfingers chocolate candy bar or a 12 oz. can of soda? a) 2 oz. Butterfingers; b) 12 oz. Coke; c) Same. I'll pick "a."

Fifth question: Fruit punch is better for you (because it has less sugar) than a can of orange soda. True or False. Again, too simple. True. This quiz is really a breeze!

The final question: Which of the following contains no cholesterol? a) eggs; b) peanuts; c) turkey. Let me think about it. I remember reading about eggs having cholesterol, so that's out. Peanuts are full of fat, so not them. Must be turkey. It's supposed to be a really lean meat. Okay, I'll go with "c."

K.C. marked her quiz and passed it to the end of the row along with her mom's and dad's papers. She figured she got them all right. Okay, she wasn't so sure about the last one, but she'd find out soon. She looked at the twenty or so people gathered in the room. All of them looked eager to hear what the nutritionist would say.

"I'm not going to grade these quizzes," the instructor announced. "The best way for you to learn is for *you* to take them back and check what you put down as I give you the correct answers."

With her paper in front of her, K.C. was astonished to find that she had missed *all* of them! "This nutrition stuff is way tougher than it looks," she whispered to her mother.

(How did you do? Answers: 1. False; 2. False; 3. False; 4. c, Same; 5. False; 6. b, Peanuts. This chapter will tell you why.)

"Let's have a show of hands," the nutritionist said. "Who got them all right?. . . Five? Four? Three? Two? One?"

K.C. glanced around the room. Only a few hands went up at first, with more raised each time the number decreased. Apparently, she wasn't the only one who thought she knew basic nutrition but really didn't.

"I see we have our work cut out for us," the nutritionist said. She smiled as she looked at each individual. "Don't worry. It's easier than you might think, given your results on this quiz. By the time you leave here tonight, you'll be equipped with the essential knowledge to make healthier food choices and help manage your weight."

* * *

Although the "class" in our vignette is fictional, we conduct actual classes on nutrition in my practice. From my patients I have learned that knowing the essentials of basic nutrition is not a given. In fact, well over 90 percent of the patients I see have no idea how the various foods we eat work to fuel our bodies. By the time you finish this chapter on nutrition, like K.C. and her companions in class, you, too, will have a basic knowledge of what foods to eat and how much.

The Information We Get Is Often Confusing

It's no wonder that nonprofessionals are confused about nutrition. So much of what we see on labels, read in magazines or newspapers, and hear on television presents conflicting viewpoints. Do we want no fat? Low fat? High carbs? Low carbs? Lots of protein? Minimal protein?

Most people believe that fat is bad so low-fat foods, by definition, must be better. But is this really true? We'll find out.

Some "authorities" proclaim that a high-carbohydrate diet is the best. In fact, you'll find many experts touting a return to the vegetarian diet that generally sustained our ancestors when meat was scarce. But turn to the next magazine and you'll find someone singing the praises of a low-carb diet. Which is correct? Stay tuned.

Some of the most popular fad diets in the past couple of decades have focused on plenty of protein, to the exclusion of carbs. Eat all the protein you want and still lose weight? Maybe for a while, but not forever? Which is factual? We'll find out.

No wonder we are confused. Even people who make a concerted effort to "eat healthy" disagree on what constitutes a healthy diet. Any bookstore's shelves groan with the weight of books on diets "guaranteed" to lop off those excess pounds, some of them even written by physicians!

It may surprise you to learn that many physicians themselves lack an up-to-date foundation in nutrition. Because in my career I have focused on weight-management strategies, I probably have a better knowledge than others, but even I continue to follow nutrition studies and consult with the nutrition specialists on my staff to continue my learning in this area. The rest of this chapter is a composite of what I have learned. I may not agree with all those diet books, but what I offer you is what works for patients in our weight management programs.

New studies are being conducted all the time. Today's knowledge of the causes and treatments of obesity can be compared with the medical understanding of causes and treatments of high blood pressure about thirty years ago. Because of massive amounts of study data over those three decades, today's doctors know how to treat high blood pressure. We hope that understanding the causes and formulating treatments for obesity won't take that long.

Let's try to brush away the cobwebs of confusion by looking at the important nutrients that make up our foods.

Six Nutrients

For the sake of ease in discussion, I have divided the essential elements we take into our bodies into six different nutrients in two basic categories. The first category—*nutrients with energy*—includes carbohydrates, proteins, and fats. The second category—*nutrients without energy*—consists of minerals (calcium, potassium, sodium, iodine, etc.—a total of twenty-two), vitamins (A, the various Bs, C, D, E, K, folate, etc.), and water.

Carbohydrates: Simple and Complex

Carbohydrates comprise the food group that contains simple sugars, complex sugars, and starches. Rice, potatoes, bread, and cereal products made from whole grains—all plant-based sources—are carbohydrates. So are vegetables and fruits, also plant-based. Carbs can also be found in dairy products and honey, which are produced by members of the animal kingdom. In a minute, we'll look at each of these carbohydrate sources in turn.

When ingested into our bodies, carbohydrates are broken down to a simple sugar called *glucose,* which is the fuel that provides direct energy to the body. Because they provide the primary fuel for the body, glucose, this group of foods should be the most abundant in our diets.

Simple vs. Complex—Way Different

The body breaks down a simple sugar quite rapidly, causing a spike in blood sugar. When the pancreas detects this high rise of sugar in the blood, it releases large amounts of insulin. It is the task of insulin to pull the glucose from the blood and get it into the cells. Because cells cannot immediately absorb large amounts of glucose, insulin helps convert the excess sugar into fat and stores it for later use. That's why we human beings get fat when we consume large amounts of simple sugars—e.g., sweet desserts, jellies, puddings—remember, it's our ancient body's mechanism for survival.

Because *complex* carbohydrates—whole-grain breads and cereals, potatoes, legumes and vegetables—tend to contain more fiber, vitamins, and minerals than simple carbohydrates, the body needs more time to digest them. This slows down the rise in blood sugar, decreasing the production of insulin. Our bodies better utilize the slowly released glucose and, therefore, do not convert the sugar and store it as fat as readily. For this reason, our diet needs to be heavier in complex carbs than in simple ones.

Complex carbs, such as cereals, can act like simple carbs in the body by removing their fiber (more about this below) and adding sugar. For example, here is the important nutrition information on General Mills' Cheerios: 1 cup has 110 calories, 3 grams of fiber, 1 gram of sugar. Three-fourths cup of the same manufacturer's Apple Cinnamon Cheerios, however, contains 120 calories, 1 gram of fiber, 13 grams of sugar. The additional apple and cinnamon flavors increased the calories (note the *much* higher sugar content) and decreased the fiber. And that's for a serving one-fourth cup smaller! That's why I ask you to check cereal labels to be sure what you're buying.

Look for Sugar Content

Remember that labels list ingredients in descending order, from the most to the least. That means, if the first ingredient is sugar, there's more sugar than anything else in that product. Sugar comes in a variety of forms, so add together all the words that mean sugar to get an idea of how much is actually in the food. What are those words? Glucose, maltose, fructose, Maltodextrin, corn syrup, confectioner sugar, brown sugar, granulated sugar. These simple sugars have been *refined* (vitamins, minerals, and fiber removed) and are, therefore, *empty* calories.

Sugar, the number-one food additive, shows up in nearly everything, including some unlikely places. Watch for hidden sugars in such foods as tomato and spaghetti sauce, pizza, bread, hot dogs, lunch meat, canned vegetables, cranberry and other fruit juices, flavored yogurt, ketchup, salad dressings, peanut butter, and fat-reduced foods. *Become a label reader!*

Fiber—Its Role in Our Diet

Our conversion of glucose into fat for storage is also slowed or halted by the consumption of fiber. *Dietary fiber* is any substance of plant origin that cannot be broken down by digestive enzymes, retaining its structure during its passage through the digestive system. This material comes primarily from the tough cell walls of plants, the part that is removed when the plant substance is refined.

Fiber, sometimes called *roughage*, is either *water insoluble* or *water soluble*, and most plants contain a mixture. Both types are beneficial. Sources of water insoluble fiber include whole-grain breads and cereals, wheat bran, and vegetables such as broccoli, spinach, and cauliflower. This type of fiber increases bulk in our bowel movements, creating easier elimination.

Fiber that is dissolved by water, i.e., soluble, includes oats, fruits, and legumes—dried beans, peas, and lentils. This type slows the emptying of food from the stomach, which helps produce a feeling of fullness (satiety). It also decreases cholesterol and carbohydrate absorption and thus helps to lower and control blood sugar and blood cholesterol levels.

When purchasing breads and cereals, look on the labels for words like "whole grains," or "whole wheat" or "whole oats." These still contain the fibrous outer cells of the grains. White bread, on the other hand, has been processed from refined flours and sugars, meaning that the fiber has nearly disappeared. Fruits and vegetables that are eaten raw contain more useful fiber than those that have been peeled, cooked, pureed, or otherwise processed. Choose fresh or frozen fruit and vegetables instead of canned. If you make your own juice at home, extract it from unpeeled fruits and vegetables if possible.

Think of carbohydrates as your energy source. But in addition to eating for energy, overweight children need to consume foods that give them a prolonged feeling of fullness and provide the minerals and vitamins required by the body. In other words, *complex,* not simple, carbs.

Types of Carbohydrates

Vegetables contain lots of fiber and vitamins but very little sugar. We can load up our diet with a large volume of veggies, feel full, and stay full longer while taking in only a few calories.

Fruits also provide lots of vitamins and fiber but do contain more natural sugar. Encourage your family to make fresh, unpeeled fruit a part of their healthy diet but be conscious of portions. Just because it's good for us, we can't load up on fruit with its high sugar content. Make small servings of fruit your family's most frequent dessert, put it on cereals at breakfast or use it as a snack in place of chips and dip.

Beans, which are actually legumes, offer us complex carbs plus lots of protein and fiber. The soluble fiber in beans helps to control appetite, decrease cholesterol, control blood sugar, and slow carbohydrate absorption. They are low in fat, have no cholesterol, and are lower in calories than other protein sources. Yes, they will create flatulence (intestinal gas), so if they have not been a regular part of your diet, add them gradually.

Starches—wheat, breads, rice, potatoes—provide a lot of energy as complex carbs. When selecting breads and cereals, read the label to make certain they contain whole grains, which include the bran. Don't forget to look at sugar content, as some cereals (remember our earlier example?) add sugar to make them tastier. For better health and weight management, replace high-sugar cereals with high-fiber ones—like bran flakes or buds and cooked oats, rice, barley, wheat, or corn grits.

Also be extremely vigilant about portion sizes. The problems arising from starches in our diets originate with restaurants that fill us up with this relatively inexpensive food. (Then we translate these portions to those we consume at home.) Protein foods tend to be more expensive, so restaurants traditionally give us immense portions of starch. We *don't need* the two to three cups of steamed rice served with a meal in a Chinese restaurant. Nor do we need massive bowls of pasta, a plate of fish and chips that is two-thirds full of fries, or cereal bowls so large they contain more than enough for two adult servings. The same goes for the dinner rolls (usually processed white bread) that we tend to obliterate while we sit and wait for the kitchen to prepare our orders.

When dining out, ask the waiter to remove the bread basket so it won't tempt your family. Eat half or less of the starches served. This is definitely a place where the idea that you should "clean your plate" should be abolished.

Dairy Products contain the sugar lactose and, therefore, are carbohydrate foods. They are also protein- and fat-containing foods. One of the best reasons to include them in our diets is the calcium they provide for our teeth and bones.

Dairy products differ in their benefits to us primarily by the amount of fat they contain. Remember the quiz in our opening scene? Question #1 was false because skim milk *does* contain the same protein and calcium as whole milk. All that is different in skim is the fat content.

To visualize the fat content of milk, try this: consider that *a pat of butter has four grams of fat and thirty-six calories.* Start with skim milk, which has only a trace gram of fat. Add to a cup of skim milk *two pats* of butter (*eight fat grams* and seventy-two calories from fat) to create a cup of whole milk, which is 3 percent fat by weight.

To arrive at 2% milk, add *1 1/4 pats* of butter to skim milk—an additional *five fat grams* and forty-five fat calories per cup. The 1% milk contains *one-half a pat* of butter per eight-ounce serving or *two fat grams* and eighteen fat calories.

Quiz question #2—2% milk is low fat, 98 percent fat free, and only 2 percent of the calories from fat—was false as well. Why? Because we're not talking about 2 percent of the *calories* but 2 percent of the *weight*. Keep in mind that the majority of the weight of milk is water—96 percent of milk's weight by volume. Manufacturers are allowed to use weight, not calories, when describing the fat percentage. Misleading? You bet! Now you know.

Simple Sugars can become a significant enemy to our children. In the past few years, the fat-free or fat-reduced craze has swept the country. What many people do not realize is that in order to maintain taste and texture, manufacturers have replaced the fat with sugar. Because we believe we're eating "healthy" fat-reduced foods, we tend to eat larger portions. After all, we're avoiding all that fat, aren't we?

The average American today eats greater than 150 pounds of sugar per year![1] Why so much? A prime cause is the replacement of milk in the diet by soda pop.

If you missed questions 4 and 5 on our opening quiz, it was probably because you have no idea how much sugar is contained in the drinks consumed in our culture. Question #4 asked whether a two-ounce Butterfingers candy bar or a twelve-ounce Coke have more sugar, or are they the same. The answer: they *both* contain the equivalent of about ten teaspoons of sugar! Likewise, fruit punch is *not* better than a can of orange soda for the same reason—they both slug 11 teaspoons of sugar into our systems. Don't we all know some kids who down three or more sodas a day, every day? That sugar volume soon mounts up.

While we're on soda, even diet sodas carry detriments to our health. The phosphorus in the carbonation present in all sodas has been found to leach calcium from bones. Studies show adolescents who drink soda instead of milk have a higher incidence of bone fractures.[2] Not only does the carbonated drink deplete calcium, that essential mineral is not being replaced by calcium from milk because teens are *not* drinking milk!

Simple sugars are present in the treats we all love. Your K.C. would surely feel deprived if she could never eat ice cream, birthday cake, or Halloween candy. I do not for a minute advise you to eliminate such treats. Such a restricted life would be no fun! Just keep them as *treats*, not everyday habits. Also control the portion size. If your K.C. loves M&Ms, let her have a single-serving size instead of buying the large economy size for the whole family to rip into. Remember, by nature we humans are completers, and we won't stop till the bag is empty!

It is not hard to eliminate from the family diet those sugars that no one really cares about. When at a restaurant, order water. I know there's a knee-jerk reaction that leads us to automatically order a carbonated beverage when we're at McDonald's. When we ask for water, the server is almost incredulous. Often, water is offered begrudgingly in a tiny cup (probably because there's no profit involved). Never mind. Just get used to ordering water as your beverage of choice. Remember that nine to twelve teaspoons of sugar (empty calories) you are saving!

When my family and I eat out, I let my children choose either a soda or a dessert but not both. I have found that it works better to let them choose how they would rather have those special "treat" amounts of sugar in their diet.

Proteins—Good and Bad

Protein foods form the building blocks of our bodies. Nearly every function of the human body requires protein in some way. As our muscles, tendons, ligaments, organs, circulatory system, immune system, skin—you name it!—slough off old cells, they need a regular supply of "fresh protein" to replace them.

To maintain health while watching your weight, it is essential to take in protein. This substance restores our muscles—all of them, including the one that is *most* vital, the heart.

As important as carbohydrates are, we *can* live without them as long as we have stored fat and adequate muscle mass. The human body can make glucose from muscles and ketones—an alternative fuel—from body fat if foods that normally provide those substances are not ingested. The same is *not* true of protein. We must eat protein to obtain specific *amino acids* that the body cannot manufacture for itself.

Amino acids come in two varieties: *essential* and *nonessential*. Of the twenty amino acids needed by the human body, nine must be provided by the diet and, therefore, are called dietary essentials. The remaining eleven are nonessential because the body can make them from remnants of leftover carbohydrates, fats, and other amino acids.

Body proteins fluctuate constantly. Not only is the protein we eat broken down to its constituent amino acids, but also the body proteins are constantly being disassembled and reassembled. In this process, called protein turnover, most of the amino acids are reformed into other, nonessential, amino acids then assimilated into body proteins. Those not assimilated or reformed are discarded and must be replaced by proteins from our daily diet.

Based on the kind of amino acids contained within them, protein foods can be divided into either *complete* or *incomplete* **proteins**. Complete protein foods contain all essential amino acids. Milk, cheese, yogurt, meat, fish, poultry, and eggs are complete. Protein from plant sources is incomplete, except for soy. With a little dietary maneuvering, one incomplete protein food can be combined with another incomplete protein food to make up for one another's deficiency. This is called complementing proteins. Check the appendix to learn how to design a meal of complementing proteins.

The body can utilize only a specific amount of protein at a time. If we take in more than the body can use at that time, that extra protein cannot be utilized for cell building and repair. It cannot be stored in the body as protein, so it is either converted to glucose for energy or to fat for storage. Eating *too much* protein, therefore, makes us gain weight.

Protein foods from meat or dairy are often high in fat, saturated fat, and cholesterol. We want to limit these three nutrients because they are associated with potentially serious problems such as heart disease, cancer, and weight gain. We should also avoid the high amounts of nitrates added in the processing of some meats. Therefore, *choose low-fat protein* foods, preferably nonprocessed.

Over the past twenty years, we've been inundated with a great deal of hype about high-protein, low-carb diets for weight loss. The premise for these diets lies with the fact that protein foods do not cause the secretion of insulin to the extent that carbohydrates do, and, therefore, people store less fat and lose weight. The supporters of such diets make insulin the bad guy, particularly because it aids in the storage of fat.

None of this is inaccurate. The problem arises when people on these high-protein diets take in *too much* protein—which can also be high in fat—causing them to gain rather than lose weight. The challenge is to get your protein as *lean* protein. A moderate intake of protein—say one to three ounces at a time—five times a day will eliminate the ravenous hunger pangs that make people reach for the quick and convenient carbs—the bagels or potato chips. Eaten in this way, the protein is used as it is taken in and not converted into fat for storage.

My clinical practice with overweight people supports the need for protein but in *small* amounts at regular intervals throughout the day. Eating unlimited amounts of protein, as advised in some of the fad diets, causes eventual weight gain. I repeat: our bodies need a small amount of protein at each meal or snack instead of a large amount at the dinner meal. No more ten-ounce steaks!

When it comes to protein intake, here's what I recommend:

1) A small amount of protein at each meal helps with satiety. At breakfast, choose a one-half serving of oatmeal with skim milk and fruit plus a boiled egg. This will prolong the feeling of fullness much longer than a sugary cereal with toast, milk, and orange juice. The latter will cause hunger to return within a couple of hours; the former will hold off those hunger pangs till noon!

2) Although those concerned about their weight generally cut down on meats with a high-fat content, anyone trying to lose weight cannot cut out protein. Therefore, make sure there is a source of lean protein at each of the three meals and one or two snacks during the day. Examples of lean protein might be one egg, two egg whites, one ounce of fat-reduced cheese, one-half cup of low-fat cottage cheese, two to four ounces of lean meat, or a combination of legumes with grains or dairy.

Because these one- to two-ounce servings at each intake are necessary for your child, work diligently to find the leanest choices. Remember that even plant protein, such as soy or peanut butter, comes with fat attached, so watch that portion control!

Sources of Protein

Beef provides a complete protein, one that has all the essential amino acids. But beef also contains fat, saturated fat, and cholesterol. Didn't we just say those can result in serious health risks? Consuming large amounts of well-marbled steaks, ribs, bacon, hot dogs, and hamburgers contributes excess calories, saturated fat, and cholesterol that can generate many diseases. Does that mean we must strike red meat from our diets forever? No.

We can keep some red meat in our diets, just not at every meal or even every day. Red meat furnishes valuable vitamins and minerals. The secret to healthier red meat lies in the selection and cooking of the beef.

Choose the leanest cuts of beef, those that contain the least fat and cholesterol. Instead of the well-marbled prime or choice, get the "select" grade of the leanest cuts: top steak round, tip round, whole round, eye of round, bottom round, or tenderloin, top loin, filet mignon, and sirloin. Make sure it is bright red in color and well-trimmed of fat.

Do not fry red meat. Instead, roast a large cut of beef (or veal) on a rack to allow the melted fat to drain away from the flesh during cooking. Cooking on a grill also allows the melted fat to drip away from the meat so that it is not consumed.

Let's talk about ground beef. Hamburgers are one of the most popular foods in our culture. Consequently, ground beef is one of the largest sources of saturated fat in the American diet today. Do you recall how you answered the quiz question about ground beef? I'll refresh your memory: "True or false, 80% lean ground beef has only 20 percent of calories from fat." That is false because, like milk, ground beef is also labeled based on weight. And like milk, water makes up the vast majority of the ***lean*** weight of the ground beef. Compared to the water, the protein and fat weigh very little. A package of meat bearing a label that shows it is 70 to 80% lean seems like a nutritional plus, since it is below the recommended amount of 30 percent of calories from fat in our daily diet. Right? Wrong. Here's what you need to understand: *the calories of the fat in the 80% lean ground beef make up over 50 percent of the total calories of the meat, making it no nutritional bargain!*

What is ground beef, anyway? It is the remains of all the better cuts of beef that have been trimmed away from the steaks and roasts, gathered up and ground together. It's an inexpensive meat for the public, a high-profit meat for the processors. If it were not desired by the consumer as ground beef, it would be made into pet food or thrown away as scrap!

Therefore, I recommend that you minimize the ground beef in your diet as much as possible. Ground turkey, I'm afraid, is not all that much better because it consists of dark meat, whose fat content is higher than the white meat turkey. When you do choose a ground beef, look for a label that says "extra lean" or displays the name "Maverick Ranch," which produces some of the leanest ground beef available—95 to 96% lean.

Pork is now being marketed as "the other white meat," touting its value as a substitute for red meat. If you choose lean cuts, such as the tenderloin and center cut chops or lean ham, pork makes a nutritious substitute for beef. Always trim off any fat around the edges of these loins and chops and definitely restrict the use of the fattier cuts of pork, such as bacon, sausage, and hocks.

Poultry should be your protein workhorse. *We highly recommend making chicken or turkey the staple meat in your household instead of beef.* The most versatile of meats, chicken is lowest in price and one of the best sources of protein without all the excess fat found in red meats. When cooked, skinless light-meat chicken is 33 to 80% leaner than trimmed cooked beef, depending on the beef's cut and grade. Chicken breast, the leanest part of the chicken, has less than half the fat of a trimmed "choice" T-bone steak. In the quantity and quality of protein, chicken compares well with beef. It supplies approximately the same amount of other vitamins and minerals, but less iron and zinc than beef.

Turkey is the leanest of meats generally available on this continent. Keep in mind, however, that the dark meat is higher in fat than the white. Be wary of turkey cold cuts, however, as they are not as lean as turkey itself. Some are made from the dark meat and some also contain organ meats—heart or gizzard—that are high in cholesterol. As already mentioned, ground turkey, often touted as a better selection than ground beef, derives 54 percent of its calories from fat, so go easy.

Fish provides not only a good source of protein but also some essential fatty acids. Choose from freshwater fish like farmed catfish, pickerel, yellow perch, trout, or the more plentiful saltwater varieties like halibut, cod, sea bass, mackerel, salmon. Some are quite lean while others contain more fat. However, the fatty fish—like salmon—provide essential fatty acids that are a necessary part of our diet. Prepare by baking or grilling rather than frying.

Eggs, although much maligned because of the cholesterol content of the yolk, can add variety to our diet. Whole eggs can be prepared poached, boiled, even baked. Egg white has no fat and can be an excellent source of complete protein. Add to salads or scramble up with salsa and vegetables for a lean, high-protein omelet.

Peanut Butter, one of the common staples of most children's diets, presents a protein source that is higher in fat content than some others but, nevertheless, offers convenience. I recommend the natural peanut butter rather than the commercial brands because it consists only of ground peanuts and salt. That's it. The oil contained in the peanut (a legume, remember) comes to the top and, therefore, must be remixed into the butter to make it spreadable. This type of fat is a healthy, unsaturated one. Most commercial brands, on the other hand, hydrogenate the natural peanut oil, turning it into an unhealthy saturated fat. Try to avoid these hydrogenated oils. (More on this topic later.)

Most supermarket chains carry their own house brand, so these natural peanut butters do not have to be budget busters.

The Good and the Bad about Fat

The third kind of energy-producing nutrient is fat. Fats and oils, although tasty, should be consumed sparingly because of their high caloric values in relation to the nutrients they provide. Fats, highly concentrated fuel, do have their place, however. We cannot delete fat from our diet, because we need it to survive! The critical key is to feed our body only the amount—and the correct type—of fat needed to function.

What are the purposes of fat? 1) It provides a source of fuel. 2) It is needed for the production of prostaglandins, hormone-like substances that regulate many body functions. 3) Certain vitamins are only fat-soluble, so without fat, we could not absorb them. 4) Fat adds flavor to foods and, because it delays stomach emptying, contains some satiety value. 5) It is needed to insulate organs, develop membranes that surround cells, regulate nerve impulses and blood pressure, assist smooth muscle contractions, lubricate the intestines, provide moisture to our skin, and help us grow hair.

How necessary is that!

Fats are classified as *monounsaturated, polyunsaturated, and saturated.* All fats contain the same number of calories per gram. One teaspoon contains five grams of fat. One gram of fat contains nine calories, so *one teaspoon of any fat contains forty-five calories.* You can see how quickly calories can add up. Carbs and protein have only four calories per gram, which is less than *half* that of fat.

In order to prevent disease, choose the healthy fats—those that are *not* saturated. Saturated fats—those that are usually solid at room temperature—come mainly from animals, except for coconut and palm oil. *These are the fats to avoid.* They can clog our arteries with cholesterol and increase the risk of heart disease. Some examples: butter, cream cheese, sour cream, whole milk, half-and-half, lard, shortening, and red meats such as bacon, beef, and lamb.

Unsaturated fats are soft or liquid at room temperature. *Monounsaturated fats, which are found in plant foods, are healthy for us and may reduce blood cholesterol.* Use these oils in cooking: olive, peanut, canola. Foods with this type of fat include peanuts, peanut butter, avocado. They are high in calories, remember, so don't eat too much of these fats just because they are "good for us"!

Polyunsaturated fats are also healthy ones, containing essential fatty acids that our body cannot make for itself. Good sources for these fats would be: seed oils from corn, cotton, soybeans, flax, wheat germ; walnuts, almonds, sardines, cod, pink salmon, tuna, rainbow trout, halibut, mackerel, herring, haddock, and flounder.

Bear in mind that polyunsaturated fats become potentially dangerous *trans-fatty acids* when converted from a liquid to a solid—into shortenings like Crisco. Manufacturers add the element hydrogen (making it a hydrogenated oil) to a liquid unsaturated fat to create a solid vegetable fat that reacts in ways similar to that of saturated fats. Remember, these are the harmful fats that we want to avoid!

Unfortunately, most of the rich desserts we love are full of saturated fat (butter) or hydrogenated oil (shortening) along with refined sugars and flour (lacking fiber).

Many crackers and baked goods are also full of those hydrogenated oils. Now that we've gone through Nutrition 101, we all know why we have to enjoy such desserts, snack foods, and crackers only rarely.

Cholesterol

Cholesterol is a fat-like substance necessary for our bodies to function. It comes from animal foods in the diet and is also manufactured in our bodies. A high cholesterol level in the blood is associated with heart disease. Changes in arterial walls consistent with deposition of excess cholesterol can be detected in children and adolescents. Believe it or not, cholesterol deposits in arteries can be seen as early as infancy! If the family has a history of high cholesterol levels, a child will be more susceptible to such deposits. So, once again, what begins as a genetic predisposition can be made worse by diet.

Concentrated sources of cholesterol include egg yolks, organ meats, fatty meats, and whole milk. We already want to limit these foods because of their fat content. Their cholesterol content gives us yet another reason.

Children need cholesterol in their diets but they will get adequate amounts from their lean protein choices. Concerns have arisen in the past that decreasing fat and cholesterol in childhood could adversely affect brain development. A recent study allays those fears: Children followed from infancy to age five were found to have no harmful effects in development from a low-fat (30 to 35 percent of calories), low-cholesterol diet.[3]

Oh, yes, back to our quiz. The final question asked which contained no cholesterol—eggs, peanuts, or turkey. Now you know the answer is peanuts, as cholesterol is found only in products of animal origin.

Nutrients without Energy

Calcium

In the body, calcium, an essential non-energy producing nutrient, gives strength and structure to our bones and teeth—indeed, to every cell in our body

Fats inhibit the functioning of calcium. The worst are the saturated fats found in dairy products (whole milk and products made with it), pork, beef, and in tropical oils such as palm and coconut. On the other hand, essential fatty acids found naturally in cold-water fish, seeds, nuts, vegetables, and botanical oils are vital to make calcium available for tissue use and to elevate calcium levels in the bloodstream.

Sugar and caffeine also interfere with the optimal functioning of calcium. Because sugar depletes the body of phosphorus—a mineral in delicate balance with calcium—if we enjoy high-sugar foods such as desserts and soda, we profoundly disturb this balance. Without this balance, calcium is not deposited to create strong bones. Caffeine can increase the risk of brittle bones because it doubles the rate of calcium excretion from the body. When the body detects that calcium is being excreted in the urine, it produces a hormone responsible for pulling calcium out of bones to maintain the blood calcium level within normal boundaries.

Maybe you think your children aren't getting caffeine because they don't drink coffee or colas. Please don't forget that many sodas (including orange and lemon-lime flavors) *add* caffeine—to boost the taste, to add a kick, and to create addiction.

Let me repeat what I said earlier: studies have shown that the substitution of soda for milk has slapped the development of our children with a double whammy—depleting the calcium in their bones and not replacing it from their diet. A recent study of teenage girls has detected greater fracture risk in those who drink frequent sodas.[4] This probably means that their bones are more brittle. If this is so, can you see how a few sodas a day for a child can lead to serious troubles for the adult that child becomes?

Excellent sources of calcium include nonfat milk, yogurt, soy milk, tofu, cheddar cheese, cottage cheese, navy beans, spinach, broccoli, kale, almonds, and sardines. Because calcium is one of the body's essentials, dairy products and vegetables, legumes, and other dietary sources of this important mineral should be included in our daily meal planning. Some of the sources—the dairy products—also contain fat, however, so don't overdo them.

Water, Water Everywhere

The minimum daily amount that an average adult should drink is eight eight-ounce glasses of water. For every twenty-five pounds a person is overweight, add another eight ounces. And that means *water*, not soda or coffee or tea or juice. *Water* plain and simple. Children, because they are smaller, don't need as much, but they need far more than most of them drink.

Why does an overweight adult need even more than sixty-four ounces of water daily? The excess weight creates a larger metabolic load for the liver trying to create energy from stored fat. The larger the load, the more water required. That's why we advise adults to drink an *additional* eight ounces for every twenty-five pounds of excess weight. For children, we tailor our water recommendation to each individual, based on that child's specific medical needs.

Why? For our bodies, which are from 60 percent to 70 percent water, this is the most important of all nutrients. It serves an essential role in nearly every function of our bodies. Water keeps the membranes of the nose, mouth, and respiratory tract well lubricated, provides form for our cells, whisks waste products from cells to the kidneys, serves as a natural appetite suppressant, and aids in digestion, which cannot proceed normally without it.

Without sufficient water, the kidneys cannot function properly. If the kidneys are not working the way they should, some of their work is done by the liver. One of the primary tasks fulfilled by the liver is to metabolize stored fat into usable energy known as ketones. If your liver is busy helping the kidneys function, you won't be able to metabolize fat and instead will store it. Therefore, the more water you make available to your body, the more fat can be burned, not stored.

A Calorie Is a Calorie—or Is It?

Does it matter whether we get our calories (energy) from proteins or carbohydrates or fats? In a word, yes. First, a little high-energy fat goes a long way; therefore, take in only a little. Second, as we mentioned earlier, a little protein at each meal prolongs the feeling of fullness, so some calories at every meal should come from protein. Third, fewer calories should come from simple sugars, especially at breakfast. Why? Because high-sugar foods lead to overeating! A study of overweight teenage boys showed that the consumption of a breakfast high in sugar induced a sequence of hormonal and metabolic changes that promoted increased food intake throughout the rest of the day.[5]

Typically, high-fat, high-sugar foods are the ones we grab for that quick, convenient fend-for-yourself meal. It does take more planning to devise a diet with low sugar and fat and more lean protein. And that's why we have so many overweight children who, if this "epidemic" isn't reversed, will become a nation of overweight adults who will severely burden the health-care system!

Learn to Read Labels

You may have picked up on our hints. We've said this half a dozen times already: read labels. When trying to put into practice what you've learned in this short course in nutrition, it is essential to read and understand the labels on the foods you buy. Of course, you now know to decrease the amount of animal fat you consume. Since we do need proteins, calcium, and fats that may have been provided by eating meat, we have to substitute other sources of these vital substances, like calcium-rich vegetables, legumes, and low-fat or nonfat dairy products. When selecting what fats to use in cooking, olive or canola are preferred. Read the labels on canned or frozen foods to determine such things as the amounts of fiber, the percentage of poly- or mono-unsaturated fat to saturated, and the amount of sugar.

Portion Control Is Vital

Now that you know what kinds of food to eat and how they work to make your body run, let's talk about *how much* to eat. We tend to be a people that goes to extremes when it comes to food, eating far more than our bodies require for fuel. When you fill your car's gas tank, would you let it run over by three or four gallons? Of course not. You fill it up and quit! When people learn to drive, they find out that if they tromp on the accelerator, shoving more gas into the engine than it can efficiently use at that moment, they waste fuel and money.

The same is true of our bodies. Yes, they need fuel—carbs, protein, and fat. But if we chomp away and give our bodies more than they can efficiently utilize at that moment, they—all together now—*get fat.*

Serving sizes are out of control. Ever notice the size of the plates, bowls, and silverware at restaurants? They're huge! And so are the food portions delivered on those plates.

Most people eat more than they need in order to fuel their bodies. Many overweight people eat significantly larger portions than necessary to fuel their bodies. We have placed a chart showing suggested serving sizes in Appendix Four. This chart is one of the most important segments in the book. You may be surprised at the serving sizes we advise. So refer to this often, until the new eating habits become well established.

When you do study the suggested serving sizes, you'll note that a Quarter Pounder at McDonald's (four ounces) uses up more than half of eleven-year-old K.C.'s meat allowance for the entire day! Its bun equals about four slices of bread, or four adult servings out of the daily allotment in that food group. Pretty easy to see how grabbing a quick burger and fries a couple times a week can sabotage a healthy eating plan!

Gradual Change, Not Quick Fix

What your K.C. needs is not a quick-fix crash diet that will take off weight in a hurry. Such diets are doomed to failure for one simple reason: as soon as dieters reach their goals of dropping ten, fifteen, twenty pounds, they typically go off the diet and return to the same habits that made them overweight in the first place. Instead, now that your whole family is equipped with the basics of nutrition, you are ready to make the kinds of changes that you can *all* adhere to for the rest of your lives.

If we are served tasty foods, we eat even when not hungry. That's just human nature. It is next to impossible to expect a child with a weight problem to muster up enough willpower to say "no" when presented with high-sugar, high-fat foods. In order to establish healthy eating habits for the child with a weight problem, the entire family must change, not just that one kid. But that's okay, because *no one* in the family *needs* all that extra fat and sugar!

Throughout this book, we provide you with easy-to-follow directions to turn poor eating habits into healthier ones. We don't expect you and your family to alter everything at once. In the first week, you might cut out unhealthy snack foods—those high in fat and sugar—and substitute controlled portions of fresh fruit, fresh veggies, or unbuttered popcorn. Increase your water intake by two; i.e., if you normally drink two glasses of water per day, go to four. The next week, go to six.

If you have always made beef your staple meat, in the second week you might try some red meat substitutes. Have beef twice that week instead of five or six times. Replace it with poultry, eggs, fish, or beans. By week three, you should be ready to cut down on portions. Again, gradual is better than all at once. If you've been accustomed to thinking that a proper serving of meat is ten ounces, cut that in half for a couple weeks. After your body has adjusted to these changes, you can go the rest of the way in cutting portions.

Gradual change is particularly recommended when increasing the fiber content of your diet. A slow, gradual substitution of high-fiber for low-fiber foods will create the least upheaval to your digestive system and will be more likely to become a permanent lifestyle change. As you start adding more fiber, be sure to increase your water intake. Otherwise, fiber can constipate rather than stimulate your system.

"But I don't like skim milk! I can't stand that natural peanut butter! Why are you making me eat this yucky fiber stuff that gives me gas?" Don't be surprised if your family gives you some attitude. That's only normal. However, remind them they have all committed themselves to strive for certain goals. Within a couple of weeks the family should adjust to the new foods and not miss the unhealthy ones from before.

Change is hard—we know. Keep at it and within a few weeks, your family won't think about it. For example, if it becomes family policy that soda is never ordered at a restaurant, then not ordering soda will become your norm—in spite of the funny looks you get from servers. If you change from a large glass of orange juice to a glass half the size, soon your family won't remember they used to drink the larger amount.

It is physically uncomfortable to be hungry, so providing foods that help your children not feel hunger will encourage them to stick to their healthier habits. Add that protein to breakfast so they won't be ravenous by ten o'clock. If the adults are out the door in a rush every morning, boil some eggs at night and refrigerate. Then your children can grab an egg for breakfast or an after-school snack, eating the whole thing or cutting it in half as appropriate.

Assuming that you are typical, even though your family commits itself to making dietary changes, you will still eat out several times a week. Be particularly conscious of healthier selections at restaurants; remember that this food is normally high in fat, sugar, and salt. Refer to the appendix for lists of healthier selections when dining out. Leave about half the food on your plate. Take it home, if you like leftovers, and enjoy yet another meal. Better yet, share one restaurant entree between two or three people.

It is important *not* to single out your overweight child at a restaurant and prohibit her from eating what the rest of the family eats. If the entire family has made the decision to eat out, then consider this one of those special treat events. *When it comes to eating, the parents set limits, deciding when and what to eat, while the children decide whether to eat and how much.* At a restaurant it's okay to be less restrictive than at home.

If the family made a choice to go out for a meal that might not be as health-conscious as usual, then the kids shouldn't be chastised for making unhealthy selections. Don't restrict your overweight child at that meal. If eating out becomes rare and special, then you can give your overweight child free rein within the family's ground rules.

If your family continues to eat out five nights a week, your overweight child may never get over her weight problem. If eating out is a necessity for your family, then the whole family, not just the overweight child, must restrict their choices. Dining out without restrictions may be fine for a special occasion, but if it's every day, you parents must take control just as you would at home. Set specific limits and do not allow the child to have free rein of the menu. Chapter 5 will tell you more about setting limits.

Chapter Recap

* Learn to select appropriate foods containing a good balance of the major nutrients—carbs, proteins, fats, minerals, vitamins, water—for meals and snacks throughout the day.

* Substitute low-fat proteins for red meat several times a week. Include small amounts of protein at every meal and snack.

* Increase intake of fiber. Gradually, please.

* Be aware that most people eat far larger portions than are recommended for optimum health and weight control. Gradually reduce portions until they reach the suggested amounts.

* Read labels. Know which fats are essential and choose those most often. Recognize that sugar goes by various names but all are still simple sugars, also known as empty calories. Be aware that percentages in meat and dairy products are labeled by weight, not by calories, so what appears healthy may be just the opposite.

* Make water your standard beverage with meals and throughout the day.

* Gradual change will meet with permanent success. Quick fixes almost never do.

Four

K.C. Tackles Exercise

In chapter 2 we looked at changes in lifestyle over the past twenty years that have contributed to the rise in obesity. We understand that when both parents work, the family dines out more often. Even when we do eat at home, often the meal is rushed so we can get on to the next item in our over-scheduled lives. We rely on convenient, prepackaged meals that can be microwaved, or fend-for-yourself snack-type foods. Some of us never manage to find the time to eat during the day, waiting till evening, when we are totally famished. Result? We take in more energy than we use, storing the excess as fat. We mentioned in passing but promised to take a deeper look at the other end of the quotient: the lack of exercise sufficient to use up the energy we consume.

More Lifestyle Changes

Until about the mid-twentieth century, people got plenty of exercise to use up all the energy they consumed just by going about their lives. Our youngsters mowed lawns, raked leaves, chopped wood for the fireplace, shoveled snow. Today, these high-energy tasks have been replaced by machines: riding mowers, leaf blowers, chain saws, snow blowers.

Much of the nation's population before the Depression of the 1930s lived on small farms. These folks stayed physically fit by doing their daily chores: mucking out stables, gathering eggs, feeding livestock, tilling the soil, tending gardens—the list is endless. As family farms fell on hard times and industrial jobs offered financial survival, more and more farmers chucked the agrarian life and moved to the city. As cities grew, they sprawled into suburbs, and the rate of normal exercise as a part of our everyday lives plummeted.

Just as our lifestyles changed in the ways we've already discussed, we've seen a major revolution in the way our communities are designed. Drive through old sections of any city and you'll see what we mean. Those communities built eighty years ago grew up with services—grocery stores, pharmacies, dry cleaners, libraries—just a short *walk* from the residences surrounding them. City dwellers back then did walk. Children walked to school, dads walked to work, mothers pushed baby carriages to the store, picked up fresh foods for dinner, returned home, and prepared nutritious meals.

When we hold weight-management seminars, I ask people in the audience to raise their hands if they walked to and from school. Most hands go up, all of them belonging to people over age thirty. Then I ask how many of your children or grandchildren walk to school now. Only one or two hands are raised. The flight from cities into suburbs and America's post-World War II love affair with the automobile changed our lives forever.

Our Love Affair with the Automobile

Today's suburban communities are planned around driving. The school bus stops out front and gobbles up our kids for a fifteen-minute ride to school. Parents must drive or ride mass transit to their places of employment many miles from home. Supermarkets, drug stores, dry cleaners, and other community services are no longer within walking distance but are gathered together in shopping centers surrounded by immense parking lots. About the only exercise we get is the short walk from the parking lot to the store. Because we seem to be forever in a hurry, we even take the parking spot closest to the door to minimize that walk.

Decline in Exercise Opportunities at School

A couple of generations ago, not only did children walk to and from school, they also engaged in vigorous exercise *at* school. Some of our older patients report that they went outdoors for recess twice a day in all but the most inclement weather. The playground equipment was minimal, requiring the kids to play active games like tag or dodge ball. Girls jumped rope, played hopscotch. Boys competed in Red Rover, a game that demanded each person in turn run hard and fast. In the higher grades, physical education classes taught organized sports like volleyball, softball, tennis, even swimming.

Over the years, however, much of this type of activity has disappeared. Some schools, fearing lawsuits from playground injuries, have eliminated vigorous outdoor activities at recess. Many school systems, hit hard by fiscal restraints, no longer budget funds for physical education classes. In fact, some high schools in poorer communities cannot afford to field school football or baseball teams, so the overall athletic program suffers. If the high school has no football team, then the junior high or middle school has no need for one as a feeder. Less emphasis on school athletic programs translates to fewer athletes at all grade levels. And fatter kids.

Never mind that kids *need* lots of physical exercise to help them grow strong bones and to consume energy so they won't store fat. That need gets lost when balanced against the *need* to fund computers and cable TV in every classroom, and— we're sorry to say, in today's more violent world—metal detectors at every exterior door.

When you were a kid, what did you do in your after-school hours? In the summer when school was out? Did you go swimming, play games, ride bicycles, roller skate, jump rope, and run around? We did. Our grandparents did. What do your kids do?

Increasingly, the answer to that last question is something like: Watch TV. Play video games. Surf the 'Net. Although we want our children to be "with it" and able to take advantage of the tremendous educational opportunities offered by the electronic age, these activities demand that our kids be stationary. Instead, they need to get up and *move*!

Television, Video Games, the Internet, and Snacks

Many Americans spend more time watching television than pursuing any other activity except working and sleeping. Over the year, school-age children spend as much time watching TV as attending school.[1] The average high school graduate will likely engage in TV watching from 15,000 to 18,000 hours while spending only 12,000 hours in school.[2] Data in this article, taken from a recent National Health Examination Survey, show that *watching TV is the most important indicator of obesity in adolescence.*

Why? First, as we've already noted, when your K.C. is sticking her face in front of the "boob tube," she is not playing energetically or engaging in sports that could help her burn excess fat. Second, while she watches TV she snacks, predominantly on foods high in calories. A recent article in the *Journal of the American Dietetic Association* reveals that during prime time television watching, the average person eats *eight times more* compared to other times of the day![3]

Watch Those Ads!

No doubt, commercials that depict mouthwatering foods being eaten by beautiful (thin!) people play a substantial role. Some evening, keep a pen and pad nearby as you watch TV. Write down what the commercials are advertising. Healthy, nutritious foods? Or cookies, doughnuts, fast-food meals? Somehow, we forget that if we eat all those foods being advertised we will look anything but thin!

During children's programming, ads are carefully created to appeal to kids. Cereal ads, for example, are not only loud and bright but also tout the taste appeal of cereal resembling cookies or candy. When we do the nutritional analysis of such cereals, we find that they are far too high in processed flour, sugar, and fat and sorely lacking in fiber and protein. From studies and from years of treating patients, we have learned that highly sugared foods stimulate more eating during the day. So if your

K.C. starts her day with one of those advertised cereals high in sugar, she'll be likely to crave even more sugar later! What a vicious circle.

TV is here to stay. So are computer games and the Internet. We wouldn't for a moment believe our patients—or you—would eliminate these from their lives. We understand that it is convenient to let the TV entertain kids while you get supper ready at the end of a hard day. And Saturday morning cartoons may help you get a few extra minutes of snooze time.

If your kids are like mine, they see those commercials for sugary cereals and bug you to buy them. Try to resist their requests, explaining that the family has made a commitment to healthier eating. Even better, see if you can substitute some good children's videos for TV programming. These usually don't have inviting commercials for cereals that are more candy than breakfast.

By the same token, we don't expect you to throw out the Nintendo and Play Station or pull the plug on the Internet Service Provider. They have their place in your lives, and that place comes right *after* the family's daily exercise!

Change in Metabolism

Your K.C.'s metabolism changes while she watches TV. Strange as it may seem, recent studies determined that children's basal metabolic rates when watching a twenty-minute TV show lapsed into that expected during a deeply relaxed, semiconscious state. Children of normal weight showed a 12 percent decline in metabolic rate, while obese children's rate declined by 16 percent.[4] In fact, the authors of this article concluded that the resting energy expenditure of the study's children watching TV was *lower* than if they were doing nothing at all!

So TV watching delivers a powerful 1-2-3 punch to children with weight problems: 1) slower metabolism; 2) increased snacking, often on the wrong kinds of food; 3) decreased physical activity.

When it comes to that 1-2-3 punch, we must also consider video games and Internet usage in the same category as TV. As the participation in these activities has risen, so have statistics on the prevalence of obesity in children and, especially, adolescents, who, like our K.C., spend much of their leisure time on the computer.

What all this amounts to is a lack of the kind of vigorous exercise our children need to burn up the energy they consume, especially when much of their diet is too high in sugar and fat. Somehow, once our children have finished their homework, written e-mails to their friends, watched their favorite TV programs—the ones their peer group will discuss in detail the next day and, as K.C. would argue, "I have to see it or be considered a total dork"—no time is left for a physical workout.

We recommend, as mentioned above, that you reverse the timing. Kids need quiet time, too. Just schedule it for *after* they walk, run, skate, jump, climb, swim.

Snacking while watching TV or surfing the 'Net is not going away. What you can do, however, is have plenty of healthy snacks on hand. Instead of chips and dip, make available apples, pears, peaches—whatever fresh fruit looks good in the market. Take a few minutes in the evening to put carrot, green pepper, and celery sticks into plastic bags, ready for the kids to munch on when they get home from school the next day. Easier yet, buy the precleaned baby carrots.

Your kids hate veggies? If you take advantage of their natural appetites when you present the vegetables, you'll have a better chance to introduce them into their diet. That's why I advise offering carrots, peppers, celery, and such for their after-school snacks, when they're ravenous enough to eat almost anything!

* * *

"Welcome, Kelly Wilkes, to Camp Timberlane." The cabin counselor looked at the list on the clipboard and greeted her with a wide smile and an outstretched hand. "Here's your name tag. Wear it for the first few days, till everyone knows everyone else."

K.C. accepted the tag, fastened it to her shirt. "I'd like you to call me K.C., if that's all right."

"Sure, sure. We aim to please. Here, take this marking pen and write your initials on your name tag." The counselor watched Kelly remove her tag and alter Kelly into K.C. before returning the marker. "Jolly good. Now, K.C., you're in bunk number five. That's the lower one in the middle, there, on the left side. Stow your clothes in the drawer marked five and your toilet articles on the shelf. Then come outside and meet your cabinmates."

K.C. did as she was told, trying to keep down the mounting excitement, palpable as a lump in her throat. She'd been looking forward to summer camp since January, when she'd persuaded her parents to let her apply. When Sara and Alexa got accepted, she knew she had to go, too. Fortunately, her application wasn't too late and here she was. She wondered if her two best friends would also be in "Harmony" cabin.

No, as it turned out, they were in "Tranquillity," two cabins west of hers. Well, she'd see them often enough in the camp activities.

That was the big selling point that pushed her parents into sending her. They all knew that the vigorous physical activity Camp Timberlane advertised was just what she needed to overcome a winter of near-hibernation. She knew she'd have plenty of chances to swim, a sport she loved. Maybe camp would also help her establish an exercise routine that she could enjoy enough to follow once she returned home. Well, that was the plan.

Orientation took up most of the first day at camp, but an hour before the dinner bell would ring, the counselors organized everyone in Junior Camp into teams for volleyball. K.C. maneuvered herself next to Sara and Alexa, in the hopes she'd be selected for their team instead of being the last one chosen, as often happened at school. It was a stupid idea, she thought later, when the counselors diplomatically made them count off by fours. That put all three of them on different teams.

Sixty boys and girls, ages eleven to thirteen, trooped off to the beach, where two volleyball nets were set up in the sand. K.C.'s team, made up of fifteen boys and girls as varied in size, shape, age, and athletic ability as one could imagine, struggled against a much superior team. K.C., who had never played volleyball, watched more than she played, trying to figure out what to do. Her teammates yelled at her. "Hey, you, get up to the net. Get your hands up. How do you expect to bang the ball back if you just stand there?" She wasn't any good, and she knew it.

Eventually, the rotation of serves came to her. Holding the ball in her left hand—she was surprised at its weight—she brought her right fist to the ball in an underhand swing, just as she'd seen the servers on the opposing team do. The ball plopped into the net and thudded to the ground. Her teammates groaned. "Put your weight into it," a skinny, pimply-faced boy yelled at her. "You've got plenty to spare."

On her second serve, K.C. could hardly see through the tears that had sprung unbidden into her eyes. She had to show them she wasn't useless. This time, she put one leg out in front and rocked back and forth between her extended legs. Then she shifted her weight to her front leg and at the same time swung her right fist under the ball. It soared over the net. She closed her eyes and prayed it would fall between the lines of players, to score a point for her team. When she opened them, to her horror she saw that the ball was coming straight for her.

"Move, move!" screamed the boy who had taunted her before. "Bend those knees. Get under it and smack it back," she heard from all around her. It was too late. The ball bounced on the ground, spraying grains of sand into her face.

When the game ended, the lopsided score was announced, too loudly, K.C. thought. A few minutes later, Sara's team defeated Alexa's team. For the second competition, the two winning teams opposed each other, while K.C. found herself across the net from Alexa, whose team, like hers, had lost their first round. "This game's too hard," K.C. complained.

"It'll get easier as you get used to it," Alexa answered as she jumped up and down in place. "You do have to move, though."

"I know. And that's hard for me."

"Yeah. Now don't go all sensitive on me and take this the wrong way, Kel, but this is exactly what you need. It'll help you get rid of those extra pounds you'd like to shed."

"If I don't kill myself first," K.C. said, trying to match Alexa's jumps with her own. During the game, her breath came in heaves as she forced her body that carried twenty extra pounds to leap and surge in pursuit of the volleyball. When it was all over, her team had lost again.

The dinner bell sounded and all sixty Junior Campers trudged up the hill from the lake to the mess hall. A few paces ahead of her, K.C. saw the skinny boy from her team in conversation with a counselor. The youngster made no effort to keep his voice down. "Don't ever put me on the same team as that fat girl, okay? This is my third year and I'm going for a ribbon in sports, but I won't be able to make it with tubs like that on my teams."

Once through the line, K.C. carried her tray to "Harmony" table. She sat on the side that put her next to "Tranquillity," so she could talk to her friends. "That was a disaster," she reported to Sara.

"Not for me. My team won. Twice."

"Yeah, well, you've always been a jock. Sometimes I wonder why I'm even friends with you."

Finished with her plate, Sara turned to her dessert of fresh fruit. "Don't get crazy on me, Kel—oops, K.C—just because you suck at volleyball. When it comes time to write the skit for Parents' Day, you'll show us all up."

"True," K.C. replied through the apple crisp she'd chosen from the dessert table, "you can run, jump, and hit. All I can do is swim . . . and write goofy stories."

"Don't beat yourself up, K.C.," Sara responded. "You're doing what your parents always wanted you to do. Your dad never was a jock, so he pushed you towards reading and stuff like that. Your mother always wants you to act like a lady and look like a model out of *Seventeen*."

"I suppose if I'm ever going to learn how to like sports, I'll just have to bite the bullet and get in there and hustle." K.C. sighed and reached for her second dessert, a giant slab of chocolate fudge cake.

"Right. We'll help. This camp will do you good. You have three weeks here to start learning," Sara said.

"And if you want to have less body to move around, it wouldn't be a bad idea to lay off those desserts."

K.C. looked at her tray, at the empty dish that once held apple crisp and at the chocolate crumbs on the cake plate. "Oh. I didn't even realize."

"No, you never do," said Sara.

* * *

Excess Pounds Limit Mobility, Emotions Elicit Unconscious Choices

K.C. has the right idea—go to camp for several weeks to get started on a lifestyle change while she's far away from her daily routine at home. In this story, she has made up her mind to change her sedentary ways into more active ones. If she can start to participate in activities that help her burn energy, chances are stronger she'll keep it up once she returns home.

Let's face it—it's very difficult for an overweight child to exercise vigorously. As our scenario shows, all that excess weight makes it tough to move! So there's a physical factor involved. When the child realizes that, as a result of her inability to move, no one wants her on their team, she will feel rejected. Now we have an emotional factor added on. And what do overweight children frequently do when they have to face an emotional problem? They reach for a comfort food to fill that emotional void. Too often, that comfort food is high in fat or sugar or both. To calm her feelings of rejection, K.C. selected *two* high-sugar, high-fat desserts—and didn't even do it consciously.

Parental Encouragement

There's yet another factor involved in our little story. Our K.C. has never been pushed to exercise. Her innate abilities lie in cerebral pursuits, like reading or writing, so those are the pastimes her parents encourage her to develop. Perhaps her parents never excelled at sports themselves so never expected K.C. to enjoy them either. Their fast-paced life affords precious little time to devote to exercise, especially if it has not been a lifelong habit. They have not set for K.C. an example of scheduling time for physical activity. K.C. is merely following in their footsteps. That's what kids do!

If we have any hope of turning around this culture's trend toward heavier, less physically active children, we have to focus on developing better eating habits *and* incorporating more exercise activities into our family lives! The kids can't (and *won't*) do it alone. Mom and Dad need to get involved.

Let me sound one note of caution here. Although we have designed this book to be a comprehensive family aid to help your overweight child (plus everyone else in the family), we do ask you to seek professional advice before starting an exercise program. Let your doctor rule out any medical condition that would prohibit your K.C.'s doing as this book recommends. That goes for you parents, too.

Our office staff includes an exercise physiologist, who develops an exercise regimen tailored to the needs of each patient registered in our weight management clinic. After I have determined the medical needs of each patient, together the physiologist and I formulate a step-by-step exercise plan to achieve specific goals. Your healthcare provider can probably help with this or refer you to a qualified professional to plan the program that is right for your K.C.—and others in the family who need to lose some excess fat.

Walk

Okay, so you don't live within walking distance of the shopping center, and you must drive many miles to and from work or school. That doesn't mean you can never walk anywhere. When you drive to a shopping center, park far away from the door and force yourself to walk. A little bit each time eventually accumulates into a useful amount. No matter where you live, you do have a neighborhood. You can start walking for several blocks—a different direction each day to vary the scenery—for half an hour a day. The whole family! Except for the purchase of a pair of good walking shoes, this exercise is *free*.

We can hear the excuses now! We've heard them all before. Too cold and snowy in the winter? Go to the mall and walk the toasty-warm indoor corridors. Too hot and steamy in the summer? Same answer. Malls are air conditioned. Don't have a residential neighborhood? Even if you live in a high-rise apartment building in the inner city, you can make opportunities to walk. Don those walking shoes and get your exercise in the hallways of your building. Walk up and down stairs instead of taking the elevator every time. No time? We can always find time to do those things that are most important to us. Yes, it takes commitment, but you wouldn't be reading this book if you weren't committed to helping your overweight child.

Believe it or not, after a few weeks of that half-hour walk—early in the morning before the day's schedule starts, or in the evening as you're winding down—your child (and everyone else who walks along) will actually discover how enjoyable it is. Not only will she be getting much-needed exercise, she may discover other benefits. Perhaps she'll get better acquainted with her neighbors as she passes by their houses or apartment doors. She can polish her powers of observation by playing sight games with family members. ("Riddle me, riddle me thee. I see something you don't see, and it's purple.") Maybe you, the parent, will use the time to review plans for upcoming days or think about work problems whose solutions have eluded you. Conversely, you might learn to quiet your mind into a semi-meditative state that eases the stresses of the day's activities.

All this and the health benefits of exercise, too!

If walking is too tame for your family and you have the money in your budget, try skating. If you choose in-line skates, remember to wear the protective helmet and joint pads. Or go bicycling. This requires even greater expense but lets you go greater distances. Many cities, recognizing the growing popularity of these sports, are installing bike/skate paths. Some rip up unused railroad tracks and convert the right-of-way to exercise paths for walkers, runners, skaters, bicyclers.

Swimming is another great way for the family to exercise together. If you don't live near a lake or ocean, a family membership at a swim club or the local Y is usually affordable. No physical activity is better than swimming when it comes to overall fitness. It exercises the entire body.

Toss the Frisbee around in the back yard. Set up a badminton net and bat that little shuttlecock back and forth. Chalk a hopscotch diagram on the sidewalk then hop yourself silly. Put some jazzy music on the CD player and dance.

See a pattern to these suggestions? They all boil down to noncompetitive sports that the entire family, regardless of age, can participate in. It may take some trial and error to discover what each family member most enjoys, but even the trials can be fun. The primary purpose is to get the family involved together, so that *the parents set an example* with their own behavior that the children will model. Both generations will be better for it.

Some family members may also compete in certain organized sports. Not only can your children develop skill in a sport, they can learn sportsmanship and "the thrill of victory, the agony of defeat." Little Leagues in nearly every town offer both boys and girls the chance to learn baseball. If you join some kind of club that provides swimming, it may also support competitive swim and dive teams. Tennis, golf, soccer, lacrosse and other sports may attract some families to build skills while burning fat and building muscle.

The only items on the family's schedule that may suffer from this commitment to exercise is the amount of time spent watching TV, surfing the 'Net, and chomping on unhealthy snacks. Good-bye, Sofa Slugs! Hooray!

Celebrate with Action, Not Eating

In chapter 2, our vignette showed K.C. celebrating with her father by eating at McDonald's. We are not totally against an occasional celebration at a restaurant. We're not *that* out of touch with reality. What we suggest, however, is to opt instead for a special *activity* to honor a significant achievement or event—an honor roll report card or a birthday. For example, how about a family weekend at a state park where every-one can hike trails, chase butterflies, look for birds, search for fossils or arrowheads? Or a day trip to a ski school? Be creative. You don't have to spend a lot; just get outdoors and walk, run, climb, swim, jump, skip, skate, bike, dance—you get the idea.

Chapter Recap

* Several factors contribute to the rise in childhood obesity over the last two decades. Our lives are more mechanized; we do fewer chores requiring vigor-ous movement, we walk less and ride more. Kids spend more time engaged in sedentary activities like watching TV, playing video games, and cruising the Information Super-Highway. Over-scheduled lives offer little time for a physi-cal workout.

* K.C., like millions of other overweight children, dislikes sports and is not good at them. Frequently the last one chosen on a team, she soothes her rejection by turning to comfort food. For her, that means high-fat, high-sugar candy or desserts. Her parents were never sports-minded and encourage her to follow more cerebral pursuits. Their lack of physical exercise becomes a role model—they don't exercise, so why should she? But she's determined to change and start an exercise routine. Summer camp—away from the bad habits she follows at home—provides her an excellent opportunity to get started.

* To help the overweight child in your family, first get your doctor's okay; then commit to "Dr. Cederquist's Family-Fun Action Program." Start walking every day. Okay, *at least* four days a week. Experiment with various types of activi-ties till you find the ones your family likes best. Opt for noncompetitive sports

to participate in together—skate, bike, swim, dance. If the opportunity and desire are present, encourage competitive sports like baseball, tennis, soccer. Parents need to teach by example. "Do as I do" always works better than "Do as I say."

Five

K.C. Bugs Her Family to Change

Ellie Wilkes was home from work and waiting in the living room when her daughter came in. "Did you have a good swim, K.C.? What did you have for lunch afterwards?" She tried to make her voice sound casual. She didn't want to sound accusatory. Before she'd left for work, she'd noticed that K.C. had started the day in one of her moods.

"The swim was great. The water was nice and warm. Before you even ask, I used plenty of sunscreen. We even met some cute boys. We left about two and had lunch. As far as that goes, I was careful, Mother," she lied. "Sara and Alexa wanted pizza, so we went to Pizza Hut, where I could get the salad."

"And did you? Did you eat just a salad?"

"No. I had the salad bar and one piece of their pizza." She knew she had wolfed down four, not one. She looked away. If her eyes met her mother's, her lie would be detected.

Ellie pressed for more information. "Swimming usually makes you ravenous. I'm surprised—but pleased—that you pretty much stuck with the salad. You've been doing so well with your eating lately."

"Yeah, I haven't had much choice with you controlling every bite I put in my mouth."

Ellie sighed. "Now don't start. You know I want what's best for you. You're such a pretty girl, and I want you to have fun in high school. You know that means slimming down in the next couple of years so you'll be popular."

"Popular! Like you were when you were a teenager, right, Mother? But I'm not like you and you know it. Look at us. Just look at the difference."

K.C. dragged her mother to the full-length mirror hanging on the back of her bedroom door. "You're a petite size six. And I . . . I don't think I wore a six when I *was* six!"

Ellie appraised both figures in the mirror. Her size six was still one size larger than she'd worn when she got married. If she watched her diet carefully and stuck to no more than 1,200 calories, maybe she could get back there. God forbid she should ever again get as large as the size eight she wore after Kyle was born! It had taken plenty of aerobics classes and a near-starvation diet, but she'd managed to return to a six. She had to admit that K.C. was right—she'd never wear a six, probably not even an eight. But her daughter would fit into a size ten by high school, if she had anything to say about it.

"Hmmm, guess you're right. You are built like your father's side of the family. Kyle's more like me."

"As he gets great joy from pointing it out to me," K.C. complained. She turned this way and that in front of the mirror. "I don't look as heavy as I did last spring, do I? I've grown a couple of inches taller, I think. All that exercise at camp and swimming three times a week this summer really has helped. And the healthier eating habits I'm developing." K.C. smiled at her reflection.

"Look at that pretty face," her mother said, "especially when you smile. I haven't seen too many smiles from you lately. It makes me happy to see you happy."

K.C. plopped down on the end of her bed and patted the comforter beside her. "Mother, can we talk or do you have stuff to do?"

Ellie glanced at the alarm clock next to the bed. "Kyle won't be home from soccer practice for a while, and you had a late lunch, so I guess supper can wait."

K.C. settled herself back into the pillows piled against the headboard. "Mother, I've tried really hard to live up to your expectations, but I need for the family to cut me some slack."

"How do you mean?"

"For starters, you can stop asking me about what I eat when you're not around. It makes me think you don't trust me."

"Can I trust you, K.C.?"

"Most of the time. But sometimes, especially after you've been watching me like a hawk at every meal, when I get away from you I go crazy and eat more than I should. I think maybe if you weren't always on me, I'd do better. You know—if I could make up my own mind about when and what to eat."

"I suppose we can try that. What else?"

"You say I've been moody lately. I guess that's true. When I went to camp, I was away from the family for nearly a month. I had lots of time to think. And I learned things about myself and the other kids and the way other families operate. We had classes about growing up, maturing—puberty—and stuff like that." She stopped, as if waiting for courage to grow within her.

"And . . . ?"

"I realized that I've always been different from the other kids I hang with. I've always known I'm smart—making straight A's, loving to read, and all that. Not good in sports. Getting my period when I was ten. And now I'm starting to need a bra. Just look at Sara and Alexa. They're not dumb, but they're not as smart as I am. They're both jocks. They don't get their period yet, and it'll be ages before they need bras. We're so different, and yet we really like each other. We're good friends. We can talk about anything."

"I'm glad you have them, K.C., really I am. With your dad away so much of the time, I have to be both mother and father to you and Kyle. I guess maybe I don't have time to talk to you as much as I should. So it's good that you have Sara and Alexa."

"It's not just that, Mother. When you do talk with me—rare as that is—you are always complaining, trying to change me, setting down rules of what to eat, how to behave. Can't we ever just have a normal conversation?" K.C. sat up, feeling brave. "Can't we ever just talk about what we're doing, things we like? Can't we set one special time when I don't have to watch every little thing I do, when you promise not to be on my case about something?"

"K.C., I'm sorry, honey. I didn't realize I did that. I . . . I can promise that. Anything else?"

"Now that I've got your attention, I have two more requests. First, when I'm trying to eat healthier foods, please don't keep stuff like cookies or potato chips and dip in the house. It's just too much of a temptation."

"That's easy enough. Done. What's your last request?"

"Make Kyle stop teasing me. It hurts enough that I'm different, and he's good at sports and apparently got all the skinny genes. . . ."

Ellie laughed and put her hand on her daughter's knee. "Now that's a tall order. But I understand. And I'll see what I can do." She stood up and ran her hands down her legs, smoothing the wrinkles out of her skirt. "I guess I do have my little compulsions. Making my daughter perfect is one of them. So please remind me when I go overboard with corrections and rules. It will take some learning—from both of us—but I promise to try."

"Me, too, Mother. Me, too."

* * *

Look at our K.C.—learning to assert herself. You go, girl!

Maybe her experiences at summer camp helped her grow bold enough to press for the changes she'd like to see. Maybe it's all those female hormones roaring through her body for the past year.

Yes, she started having her period—the medical term is "menarche"—at the age of ten. Although you may think that's *way* early, ten is only a little early. Over the last century the age of menarche has moved up from age fourteen to more like late eleven or twelve, generally as a result of better nutrition. However, we have found that puberty is accelerated in overweight children. Girls need a certain amount of body fat for menstruation to occur. For someone overweight—like our K.C.—menarche at ten is not unexpected.

Having her periods when her best friends haven't started yet makes K.C. different in yet another way. We wanted to make clear that the overweight girl who goes through puberty earlier than her peers must deal with a whole host of issues. Not only does she get teased for being too heavy, she may also feel uncomfortable around her friends when she's menstruating and they are not. Then she can anticipate early breast development, the need to shave armpits and legs—all necessary to help her fit in. Remember, the last thing an adolescent ever wants to be is *different*!

Yet, K.C. can still be on her way to becoming a well-adjusted young woman, able to assert her needs and ask for the family to cooperate in meeting them. This type of interaction is not unusual within a healthy family relationship.

Lots of family stuff goes on in this little story. We created this scene to give us a chance to talk about how families operate, especially as these "family systems" relate to problems of weight management. We won't get too technical but will use some of the terminology that you might encounter if you should ever talk with a family counselor or read family therapy self-help books.

Family Systems—Enmeshed or Chaotic

The interrelationships of family members run the gamut from those that are so closely interwoven as to be considered "enmeshed" to those that are so disengaged as to be termed "chaotic." These are extremes. Most families exhibit healthier relationships, falling somewhere in between.

The Wilkes family, as we have created them for the purposes of this book, are borderline "enmeshed." The mother, because she is the only parent around most of the time, has become overprotective. She does "watch her like a hawk," as K.C. complains in our vignette. From long experience, K.C. knows that her mother wants to hear all the details of her activities—not just what she ate for lunch when not in her presence, but whether she used sunscreen, and even if K.C. might have engaged in some harmless flirtations. K.C. longs for her mother to see her as an individual with her own needs separate from her mother's, and manages to work up the courage to confront her with some requests for significant change.

How an Overprotective Atmosphere Relates to Weight Problems

Some of the patients we see in our office come from this type of overprotective, too closely involved atmosphere. Many tell us that throughout their childhood, they cannot recall a time that they have not been "on a diet," or when their hands were not being figuratively slapped every time they slipped a morsel into their mouths. Someone else always sets the parameters about when, what, and how much to eat, so they never learn to listen to their body's needs and regulate their own dietary intake.

Like K.C., such children rebel from these constant dietary constraints by eating too much or the wrong kinds of food when away from the controlling parent, even though they know better. This emotional response is typical of children, no matter what kind of family system they live in.

How a Chaotic Atmosphere Creates Weight Problems

On the other hand, we also see overweight patients who come from families that are too disengaged, nearly to the point of having no interaction. In these "chaotic" interrelationships, members of the family function more independently of one another. Often, no one is really aware of anyone else's day-to-day lives. Few guidelines or rules exist; rather, all—parents and children alike—are off doing their own thing. Because parents don't communicate closely with each other, they often send mixed signals to their children. The parents might be dealing with marital or substance abuse problems, either of which can cause stress in the family. Stress often results in overeating, to fill the emotional void.

Both parents in this type of family may be extremely wrapped up in their work and never establish designated family times for meals. As soon as they are old enough, the children must fend for themselves with regards to food, with no consistent limits of any kind. The children learn very few guidelines on what constitutes a meal and are free to eat chips or pizza or candy every day.

In such a chaotic environment, children are typically unable to self-regulate their eating behavior. They eat whenever food is present, probably out of an unconscious fear stemming from the fact that food has not been provided with any degree of consistency. Their thought process seems to be: I have to eat it now, when I can, because it might be gone the next time I'm hungry.

No "Perfect" Families

Perhaps you recognize some issues that apply to your own family, perhaps not. I doubt that there is any such thing as a "perfect" family, one that demonstrates no elements of being either enmeshed or disengaged. My point is that all families can profit from being open to change, especially the positive changes that we know can be effective in managing a weight problem.

How to Improve Family Interactions

The first step, as shown in our vignette, is to face the realities of a situation. Here, K.C. gathered up her courage enough to make some requests of her mother. She started with three:

1) Let's open our communication so that when we talk, it's not always about rules and behavior. 2) Keep unhealthy foods out of the house so I won't be tempted [especially when no one is around to monitor me]. 3) Get everyone in the family [even that pesky little brother] not to bug me.

Underlying all of these requests is the need to take more responsibility for her own actions. K.C. is, after all, growing up and needs to feel that her decisions can be trusted. But first, she must be allowed to make those decisions herself.

Parents' Responsibilities

Most children do not shop for the family's groceries. The parents do that. Most children do not plan, prepare, and cook the meals. Parents do that. So let's start with some responsibilities for parents who want to help their overweight child.

By this point in the book, you are familiar with the appendix. Using the "Food Choices for Good Health" that you have no doubt discovered there, before you head for the supermarket, make a list of food items to shop for. Write on your calendar the meals when your schedule will permit the whole family to dine together and what meals the children will need to make for themselves. Be sure to keep healthy snack items on hand, not just for the child with the weight problem but for everyone in the family. It really isn't fair to the overweight child to keep tempting foods in the house then blame the poor kid for wanting to eat them when everyone else does. The family does not always have to be "on a diet," but it is important to make a conscious effort to limit empty calories in the family's diet.

As you learned from Nutrition 101 in chapter 3, for desserts and snacks, choose fruit instead of pastries; veggies instead of chips. Peaches, pears, apples, grapes and other fresh fruits provide better nutrition and less energy than cookies, chips, or candy, even the reduced fat kind. Remember that prewashed baby carrots, celery, and green peppers cut into strips make excellent after-school snacks and, when introduced at the time kids are hungriest, teach them to eat such vegetables. If at first they balk at snacking on veggies without dip, the appendix contains some recipes for low-fat dips you can easily make at home.

Make a commitment to introduce healthier eating habits to your family. Some we've already talked about, such as eating more slowly and in only one or two designated places. Let me now suggest a few more easy-to-make nutritional changes that can result in a big difference in energy intake.

Fruit Instead of Juice or Flavored Drinks

Always choose the fruit itself over a fruit juice or a fruit-flavored drink. Fruit promotes a feeling of fullness, while juices are quickly metabolized and soon leave your child hungry again. Juices, even those that are 100 percent juice, lack the fiber that is important in digestion and satiety. Beware those fruit-flavored drinks that advertise they "contain 100 percent of the day's requirement of vitamin C." Typically, these drinks are pumped full of sugar. It is easy to drink large quantities of these fruit-flavored, sugary drinks to quench thirst and, at the same time, add many calories.

Water Instead of Soda Pop

If your family has always made soda pop a staple of your diet, let me suggest once again that you make these only *occasional* drinks instead of your everyday beverage. Soda offers no nutritive value; its calories are "empty." Instead, replace soda pop with water as the staple beverage of the household. Changing this habit is a nearly painless way to avoid extra, non-nutritive or "empty" calories.

Skim Rather Than Whole Milk

Did I mention milk? Let's talk about that. As a family physician as well as a bariatric physician, I know that even the most conscientious parents have incorrect information about the kind of milk to feed their children. Younger than two, children need to drink whole milk for important brain development. However, after the age of two, the only benefit children get from whole milk is excess fat—something most do not need.

Don't be confused by food labels. Many parents think that 2% milk is a low-fat milk containing half the fat of whole, or 3%, milk. They figure that a liquid that is 98 percent fat free should be a nutritional bargain. Wrong.

Let me review what you already learned from chapter 3: Whole milk contains *eight* grams of fat per cup; 2% milk contains *five* grams of fat per cup. On the other hand, skim—or fat-free—milk contains *no* fat but *all* the protein, carbohydrate, and calcium of whole milk. Therefore, *I recommend skim milk for the entire family above the age of two.* Children reared on the taste of skim milk become accustomed to it, whereas those raised on whole or 2% milk may find skim milk watery if introduced to it later in life. No matter when you provide skim milk to your family, they *will* become accustomed to it within a few weeks.

Hints to Relieve Stress of Meal Preparation

I encourage families to take advantage of modern conveniences, such as the prewashed baby carrots that need no further preparation and frozen vegetables. Broccoli bits or vegetable medley in frozen packages provide as much taste and nutrition as the fresh variety, perhaps more if fresh veggies are not used before they pass their prime. Their quick addition to a fast meal like baked chicken breast—or even pizza—help round out the meal's nutritional value. Prepare foods ahead of time. One way is to double your recipes when making casseroles, lasagna, meatloaf, and the like, and freeze half to be used later. Use quick cooking methods such as the microwave or pressure cooker.

Summary of Other Parental Responsibilities Previously Discussed

As noted before, parents also carry the responsibility to schedule regular mealtimes and make a concentrated effort to eat together as a family as often as busy schedules permit. If dinner is out of the question, at least get together for breakfast. To avoid the early morning rush, set the table the night before.

Parents should establish one or two designated areas for dining, such as the kitchen and dining room, *not* in front of the TV or computer. Together, family members can plan meals and snacks before each trip to the supermarket. Preplanned menus can relieve some of the stress of mealtime preparation. Whoever serves the food is responsible to tailor portion sizes to the differing needs of each family member and to serve from the stove rather than from large bowls on the table. The latter promote second helpings.

Parents need to be careful to establish fun, pleasant conversation at mealtimes. Never should meals be a time to bring up problems children are having, to correct their behavior, or to harangue them about schoolwork, grades, uncompleted household chores, etc. Make it a time for all family members to share what's going on in their lives. Promote a positive, stress-free environment at the table, keeping in mind that many children overeat as a result of stress.

These family-centered changes all fall onto the parents' to-do list. What should the child be responsible for?

The Child's Responsibilities

First and foremost—and perhaps the most difficult change for the parents to allow—children need to be responsible to decide when they are full. That means *they do not need to clean their plates!*

No More "Clean Your Plate!"

I realize that this advice flies in the face of family tradition. The idea that you had to clean your plate may have begun during the Great Depression, when food was scarce for much of the population. Wasting even a morsel was tantamount to a crime! Probably the seniors in your family tell tales of times when they would gobble up anything left on the plate by someone else in the family. I know I've heard such stories from my grandparents.

Or maybe the "clean your plate" imperative came as a result of widespread famines in various places in the world. One of my patients remembers it as "Clean your plate; remember the starving people in China." Another recalls it was the "starving Armenians."

Perhaps the admonition came as a way to force kids to eat strange foods still too sophisticated for their child's palate. "Clean your plate or you don't get any dessert," prodded many a child to whisk away unsavory foods—not always into their mouths, but maybe to the family dog waiting expectantly at their knee.

If one of the goals for any child with a weight problem is to learn to stop eating when she recognizes that her body has had enough, then it is counterproductive to insist that she clean her plate. So please, if you have been insisting on this, *stop.*

Allow Child to Decide What to Eat

Second, let the children determine not only how much, but what they will eat. It is not necessary for all people to like all foods. Until a child's tastebuds are fully developed, some foods just won't taste good, and some foods might even make the poor kid gag! So, do not hesitate to introduce a new, healthier food but allow the child to nibble it and decide whether to eat it or not. If they are not ready yet to enjoy its taste or texture, wait a few months and try it again. In time, it might even become a favorite food—*if* you don't force it on them before they are ready. A food should never be used as either punishment or reward (since you ate that candy bar at the movies this afternoon, you can't have any strawberries tonight; *or* if you eat the zucchini, you can have some chocolate cake).

Let the Child Refuse to Eat

Third, let your children refuse to eat. Maybe they just aren't hungry. If they aren't, don't worry. That's normal. Just wait and offer food at the next meal or scheduled snack. When they're hungry, they'll eat.

Don't Force Child to Report Everything Consumed

Finally, if appropriate for the age of the children, allow them to choose what they eat when parents are not around and *not have to report back*. If the family is committed *together* in their desire to follow healthier eating habits, then trust the child to make good decisions most of the time. Everyone slips from time to time, but the more trust placed in your children, the better they will live up to the healthier expectations and limitations they have helped to formulate. An *occasional* cookie or piece of cake will not hurt your child. Forever forbidding certain foods can do harm, as they become more desirable. Remember that the old saying "forbidden fruits taste sweeter" applies to your family's eating habits.

Build Your Child's Self-Esteem

Trusting your children also helps to develop their self-esteem. In our scenario K.C. didn't tell her mother the whole truth about what she ate *this time*. But she also recognized her mother's constant harping as the cause of her own rebellion. K.C. then asserted her needs and asked that they be met by others in her family. To do that requires self-esteem. A child learns to value herself when she understands that others value her as an individual. Trusting the decisions your children make tells them you value them as individuals who have desires and needs separate from yours.

Even though Mrs. Wilkes is overprotective and has her own agenda for K.C.'s development—i.e., she wants K.C. to become thinner not only because it's healthier but so that she will be "popular" when she gets to high school—she listens attentively when her daughter has something important to talk about. That fosters self-esteem. She doesn't tell K.C. she's off base but instead affirms the validity of what she requests. That generates self-esteem. She promises to try to make happen what K.C. asks for. That creates self-esteem.

In her responses to her daughter's requests, Mrs. Wilkes is giving her unconditional love. That, most of all, promotes self-esteem.

Open Lines of Communication to Resolve Family Conflicts

The story also demonstrated that, when love and understanding are engaged, it is possible for a child to open up to a parent and share her feelings, desires, even fears. Let's not forget that parents often erect formidable barriers to free communication with their children. After all, Mom and Dad are the authorities in the family. Usually what they say goes. A child has to be pretty strong to break down some of those natural barriers and express her needs. Unless the parents invite children to talk about their feelings in a nonjudgmental atmosphere and promise to resolve conflicts in a reasonable, non-threatening way. That means no yelling, no denials, no faultfinding. Some families have never experienced this type of atmosphere and don't even know it is possible.

It can be a beautiful, loving journey of discovery.

Chapter Recap

* K.C., operating in a fairly healthy family system, becomes bold enough to lobby for some much-needed changes that will improve her chances of meeting her weight-management goals.

* Families may show elements of being "enmeshed"—too closely involved and overprotective—or "chaotic"—disengaged to the extent that the kids are pretty much on their own. Most, however, fall somewhere in the middle of the spectrum.

* Family interactions, especially as related to helping the overweight child, can be improved with commitment and cooperation. First, the parents need an understanding of their responsibilities in conjunction with initiating healthier eating habits. Their job entails shopping for healthy foods, to keep them available in the house for meals and snacks, especially when the kids have to fend for themselves. They need to substitute fruit for juice, limit soda pop to occasional usage, and make water the primary beverage of the household. Instead of whole milk, they should introduce skim milk as soon as the child reaches the age of two. Parents determine when to offer meals and snacks, what foods to serve and where to eat. Together with their child, the parents then establish what the child is responsible for. This includes whether to eat, which of the offered foods to consume, and when to stop. Once the child becomes aware of the need for healthier eating habits and selections and tries to comply, the parents need to trust the child and not force her to report food consumed out of their sight.

* Of primary importance to this process is the building of the child's self-esteem, through trust, validation of her needs, and unconditional love.

Six

K.C. Faces a Crisis

"You know, seventh grade hasn't been that tough so far," K.C. announced to Sara as they rode the bus.

"Not for you, maybe. You always get straight A's. And sometimes without even cracking a book."

"Yeah, in elementary school, but now school is much harder."

"Right. And didn't you just a second ago tell me that you don't think it's so tough?" Sara watched as K.C. flushed. "I rest my case."

The first five weeks of the fall semester had been a breeze, K.C. realized. During the summer she and her friends had shared their ideas about what to expect—getting lost in the cavernous hallways of the much larger middle school, changing classes every hour, not allowing them to get to know one teacher really well as they always had at Park Place School, harder courses, tougher grading standards. Then, of course, there would be all those cute boys from the other feeder schools, boys they'd never met. How distracting was that!

Actually, K.C. was surprised at how well she'd adjusted to everything. With her mother's help, she'd managed to establish a pretty effective after-school routine. As soon as she got home, she'd munch on veggies or fruit and wind down from the day's school activities with a few minutes on the Internet. Then, for an hour before supper, she would exercise. Most often, she'd walk. Other times, she rode her bicycle around the elementary school track. After a quick shower and a pleasant dinner with Mom and Kyle, it was time to hit the books. Once she'd completed her homework and her mother had checked to be sure she did all the assignments, she could watch her favorite TV programs till her 10:00 P.M. bedtime. The alarm got her up at six for ten minutes of jumping rope then a good breakfast—usually oatmeal, fresh fruit, and yogurt or scrambled eggs (mostly the whites), dry whole-wheat toast, and skim milk— then a brisk walk to Sara's home three blocks away to wait for the bus. She was closing in on her weight and exercise goals and looking *totally awesome*. Yes, she felt really good about her progress in seventh grade.

"How tough do you think our six-weeks' tests will be?" Sara's question brought K.C. back from her thoughts.

"Oh, not so bad if you've been working all along. Pretty awful if you've left all the studying till now."

"Well, Miss Efficient, we can't all be like you."

"Sara, don't worry. You're smart and you've been studying. In fact, we've studied together sometimes, so I know you'll do fine. It's Alexa I worry about."

Even though she lived only a few blocks away from their neighborhood, Alexa had to take a different school bus, so the three of them now saw each other mostly on weekends.

"Me, too." Sara shook her head. "We've got to work on that girl. She's been totally weird lately. Why don't we set up a study time together Saturday and review with her for some of the tests."

"Saturday morning. Don't forget, the afternoon belongs to Daddy.

"How could I forget? You've been having your Saturday matinee date with your father for as long as he's been on the road." Sara grinned, trying not to look envious of the fun times K.C. always had with her dad. "I'll call Alexa and set it up. Nine o'clock at my house?"

"Perfect. We won't have Kyle to pester us there. An hour each on math, English, and social studies, and I'll be home for lunch before my afternoon date with Dad."

At 8:30 Saturday morning, K.C.'s phone rang.

"Hey," Alexa said. "I wanted to get you before you left for Sara's."

"Oh? What's up?"

"I can't make it. We'll have to cancel our study group."

"Why? Are you sick?"

"No, it's nothing like that." Alexa's voice sounded secretive, evasive. "I'll explain later."

"How about tomorrow afternoon? After my family and I get home from our swim at the Y?"

"Maybe. We'll see. Call me when you get home, okay?"

K.C. stared at the phone in her hand until the long dial tone turned to staccato off-the-hook beeps. Something was going on with her good friend.

What would she do now, with three hours of unscheduled time before her date with Dad? K.C. wondered. She ticked off her options: do some studying of her own, walk for an hour then surf the 'Net, watch the movie her mother had rented yesterday. She'd exercised enough this week, she figured, and studying could wait till Sunday. She shoved the video tape into the player and settled into the recliner.

Two hours later, her father walked in just as she hit the rewind button. "Hey, K.C., was that a good one?"

"Not too bad, but more Kyle's speed than mine."

"Probably because your mother planned to watch it with him while you and I were gone this afternoon."

K.C. grinned. "Yeah. I checked the newspaper. The movie I want to see starts at 1:20."

Bill Wilkes eased his bulky body onto the sofa and leaned toward his daughter. "I have to talk to you about that, sweetie."

A prickle of fear brushed the back of her neck. "Why?"

"Something's come up. I can't make our date today. I have to meet with a very important customer who came to town yesterday. My boss just phoned to demand my presence."

"All afternoon, or could we make the four o'clock showing?"

Her father sighed and took her hand in his. "Afraid not. No telling how long this might last. I'm sorry, babe, but we'll just have to let it go for today."

K.C. fought back tears. "I thought our date was never to be interrupted for anything. You promised."

"Yes, and this is the first time in several months that I haven't made it. Isn't that right? Don't I usually keep that promise?"

"Usually. But I really looked forward to today. It's been a tough week and I wanted to tell you about it. And Wednesday was my twelfth birthday and you weren't here to celebrate it with me. We were going to do that today."

Bill stood up. "K.C., I called you from Chicago on your birthday. Aw, honey, you know I wouldn't break our date if it weren't absolutely necessary. This is a huge account, and I can't afford to upset this guy—or my boss. I have no choice."

"Yes, you do, and you choose them over me."

"K.C., that's not fair. Please don't get so upset. Why are you so angry?"

K.C. let her rage overwhelm her. "Because I am, that's all. You're never home during the week. You give all week to your work and on the weekends it's supposed to be family time. *Our* time."

Bill sat down again and silently stroked his daughter's arm till she calmed down. "Sometimes grown-ups have to do things they really don't want to do. My job is important—to me, to the whole family. When my boss says, 'Be there,' I have to go. That's just the way it is, K.C. It'll happen to you someday, when you're a grown-up. And you'll remember this day and understand."

"I don't want to be a grown-up if it means breaking a promise to my child."

Bill slowly rose to his feet, trying to hold onto his patience. "I've already apologized for that. Now, you'll just have to get over it." He pulled K.C. into his arms but she backed away. "Too grown up for a Daddy hug?"

"No, too mad." K.C.'s feet punished the floor as she huffed off to her bedroom. She dropped onto the bed and folded her arms across her chest. First, Alexa broke their study date. For no reason. What's up with that? K.C. wondered. Now her dad had to work instead of taking her to the movie. To top it off, she just started her period, so there'd be no swimming with the family tomorrow. It was just too much.

Sunday morning, when Ellie Wilkes vacuumed under K.C.'s bed, she found the remains. Three packages, all empty: a box of chocolate chip cookies, a giant bag of peanut M&Ms, and what looked like—yes—Twinkies. She shook her head. Her K.C., who had been doing so well for so long, had gone on a binge.

* * *

Why K.C. Went on a Binge

Well, it was going to happen sometime—a major disappointment or a combination of several stresses would test our K.C.'s commitment to her healthier habits. First, she worries about one of her closest friends, who shows signs of having some unknown problem. That's a very normal thing for a child of twelve to do! Second, it's exam time and even though she's a good student, she feels some anxiety. Third, her father couldn't make their appointment, a time she cherishes, especially *this* week. And finally, she has her period.

K.C. is only a child, after all, and even adults can have difficulties sticking to their resolve when a crisis occurs. So she went on a binge. Is it the beginning of the end? Will she regress and undo all the progress she's made?

No.

Use Relapse to Show Unconditional Love

Relapse happens. Don't go crazy when it does. Talk with your K.C. Reinforce all the good habits she has worked to establish and don't dwell on the relapse. In fact, when a crisis like this happens, you can view it as a prime opportunity to demonstrate your unconditional love. Give her positive messages: "Honey, I'm not in the least bit mad. You did what anyone would do, even me. You are getting so close to the goals you set for yourself, and I'm so proud of the progress you've shown over these months. I know you won't let this little falter bother you but will get right back to your healthier habits."

Keep your own disappointment under wraps. Don't blame, accuse, or punish by saying something like: "Look at all the junk you ate just because you were mad. That was stupid. Don't ever do that again." Now is a time for understanding, not condemnation.

This binge, like most of them, was born out of the need for emotional nourishment rather than out of physical hunger. K.C.'s eating all that junk food resulted from an unconscious desire to numb powerful emotions, emotions that she, a child, has not yet learned how to handle. All people, not just those with weight problems, have emotional urges. However, using food to respond to those urges is more typical of overweight people.

Hidden Reasons for Overeating

Let's look at some of the hidden reasons people might eat. One of the hidden reasons for eating isn't all that hidden. Sniffing, tasting, chewing, swallowing food—these are all pleasurable experiences. By nature, we enjoy eating. And we don't enjoy the feeling of hunger. Hunger, a very strong drive, was built into our bodies as a survival mechanism. When hungry, a baby lets us know by crying. A child's plaintive "I'm hungry!" can cause the most determined driver to pull off the interstate and into a restaurant.

Moreover, tasty foods are everywhere, tempting us to overeat. Long gone are the days of bland diets of basic meat and vegetables. Our supermarkets—and our refrigerators—are full of delicious goodies. We are surrounded by tasty choices so we can turn down anything we don't absolutely love. And when we absolutely love a food, some of us go overboard and eat more of it than we should.

Anger, Boredom, Stress

Anger comes pretty high on the list of hidden reasons for eating, as our little story shows. K.C. hasn't learned how to express her anger, or even that it's appropriate to do so. She may have started out being angry at her father, but later she may have turned that anger toward herself. Some children believe that they are not supposed to get angry at their parents so when they do, they also feel anger against themselves. They are ready to learn that the constructive expression of anger is healthy, far healthier than keeping it bottled up inside or exploding it in a bout of gobbling down every morsel short of roadkill.

Boredom ranks right up there with anger as a cause of emotional eating. Our K.C. had time to fill, several hours of time she thought she would spend with her dad. Some children feel that they have to be productive in every moment of their lives. They *must* be doing something constructive at all times or the consequences will be feelings of inadequacy. They think: "I'm not good enough so I'll demonstrate my worth by keeping busy and productive." They view eating as a productive activity, and once they start, they find it hard to stop.

You, as the parent, need to help them learn that it's okay to relax, to have some down time, even to be self-indulgent with relaxation occasionally. Teach them that it's just fine to lie on a blanket in the front yard and watch clouds go by, or laze away several summer hours searching for a four-leaf clover or shells on a beach. In fact, do it with them!

Another hidden reason for eating would be stress—anxiety, especially over something beyond the person's control. K.C. feels anxious not only about her own upcoming exams but also about what she assumes is a problem for her friend Alexa, a situation over which she has no control. She's in the dark, out of the loop, and nervous. So she eats.

Family Secrets

Some of the overweight children we treat in our office are reacting to a family stress. In some cases, one of the parents is gravely ill—facing cancer, recovering from a heart attack—and the child is "saved" from knowing the details by well-meaning relatives. Kept in the dark about something she *knows* is going on, she eats. Or the parents are contemplating divorce and keeping that possibility a secret. The children feel the disharmony, sense the probability of a marital breakup, and the anxiety of the situation pushes them to eat. While the parents are dealing with the breakup, they have little time or emotional reserves to spend with the children, so the kids fill that void with food.

Fear

Anger, boredom, anxiety and—let's not forget—fear. Some psychologists feel that only two emotions affect our behavior: love and fear. Fear, they suggest, lies beneath all other emotions that are not love. Anger isn't really anger, it's fear in disguise. K.C.'s anger at her father might be, instead, fear that she doesn't measure up to his expectations. Fear of rejection is the true emotion that jumps out in the form of rage.

Fear that if you don't do something important every minute, you won't be loved. Fear that the sick parent may die. Fear that after the divorce, you will be lonely, impoverished, forgotten by the noncustodial parent. Powerful emotion!

Some children actually fear a parent. In this less-than-perfect world, some kids live in an abusive family and feel that if they eat, they'll make themselves bigger, more powerful. Or less desirable. (More about this later.)

It's Prudent to Seek Professional Help

In times of crisis, it is easy to get overwhelmed by emotions. I frequently recommend that my patients in crisis turn to family therapists for assistance in handling these difficult situations. Understand that seeking professional help carries no stigma. It's the prudent thing to do, to learn how to handle the crisis in the healthiest manner possible.

Learning to Recognize Hunger as Physical or Emotional

Emotional hunger may feel the same as physical hunger if you don't know the signs to look for. Your K.C. can learn whether she is truly hungry or using food to fill an emotional need. The best way to learn the signal of hunger is to allow some time to elapse after first thinking of eating. If your K.C. feels, "I'd like to eat," teach her to put the food down and turn on a kitchen timer. Wait three minutes. If she still wants the food when the timer sounds, she can eat it. Chances are strong that if the urge was an emotional one, it will have disappeared in the three-minute wait.

Influence of Family and Friends

Besides emotional urges and hidden reasons, encouragement by friends and relatives pushes children to eat when they shouldn't. In most households, food equates with love. Haven't we all visited a friend or relative who insisted we eat something, even if we weren't hungry, and a "no thank you" would be not only ungracious but downright unloving? Remember the annual family reunion when Great-Aunt Sylvia invariably makes her famous German chocolate cake because she knows how much your K.C. loves it? How could she refuse the gigantic piece of cake Aunt Sylvia slaps onto her plate?

Holidays can often present difficult decisions. Many families overeat at holiday dinners, sometimes several days in a row. Knowing these times are approaching, you and your K.C. can sit down and plan in advance what she will and won't put on her plate. Have fruit treats on hand for your K.C. to choose instead of cookies or cakes. Instead of baking holiday treats, the family can have fun making non-edible crafts and gifts.

Then there's the birthday party your K.C. goes to for her best friend. How could she push aside ice cream and cake when everyone else is chowing down? She doesn't have to refuse. The occasional piece of cake—even one the size of a dinner plate—won't wipe out months of healthy eating. An important part of life with family and friends is to do whatever the others are doing. We don't want our K.C.—or yours—to feel left out.

When your child first starts watching what she eats, she may have a tendency to go overboard at such times. However, as discussed before, she will soon realize that no one will stop her from having all she wants and, consequently, she is less likely to overeat.

Try role playing with your K.C. to help her learn how to manage relatives or friends who might push unwanted food on her as a means of expressing affection. She can learn some phrases to use to help them understand how she feels. "Gramma, the kids teased me about my weight, and I couldn't do all the activities I wanted because I was too heavy. So I've been trying to exercise and eat healthy foods. I'd really love it if you would help me stop eating high-sugar or high-fat foods." Most relatives, asked in this way, would cooperate.

Wise Words for Relapse Management

You can expect relapses. They don't mean you or your child have failed. So don't be too hard on yourself or your child. Use a relapse as a teaching experience.

Parents of an overweight child who experiences a binge can help the child learn how to deal with her feelings. Let me suggest a few words of wisdom you might like to share with your child.

First, let them know that emotions are not to be ignored or turned off. Encourage them to acknowledge the fear, boredom, anxiety, or anger that fostered the binge. In our K.C.'s situation, she might say, "I'm afraid Alexa has a serious problem and I don't know what it is." Or "I know—really I do—that Daddy had to see that important customer, but I was hurt that he didn't tell his boss he couldn't and instead choose me."

Next, remind them that food cannot solve their problems and, in the long run, may create even more. They know. Help them to affirm it with words. "I wasn't really hungry for the cookies or the Twinkies. I recognize peanut M&Ms have always been my comfort food, but I'm ready to find comfort in something else. Instead, I'll take comfort in the fact that I'm slimming down and much closer to the body I'm supposed to have."

Constructive Alternatives to Eating at Time of Emotional Need

Finally, suggest alternatives to food that may help them deal with emotions. One of my patients cleans her dresser drawers or rearranges her closet any time she feels emotionally vulnerable to overeating. In her goal journal, she made a commitment to replace emotional eating with activity. Not only does the activity give her a chance to clear her head about the sequence of events that pushed her to the edge, but it also allows her to do something constructive. She has the neatest drawers and closet in her household!

Prevention Better Than Cure

Prevention is within your reach. We in the medical community constantly hammer at prevention because preventing disease is so much better than treating it after it happens. With the information provided by this book, you can prevent your overweight child from continuing the cycle and becoming an overweight adult. If *all* today's overweight children turn into obese adults, the stress on our health system in a few years will be immense! The increased incidence of diabetes, circulatory system disease, cancer and other debilitating illness would devastate our already overburdened medical community. I don't even want to think about it!

The critical time to conquer weight problems is now, before your child becomes a teenager. It's not even too late then. Keep in mind, however, that by early adulthood, eating and exercise habits (or lack of them) are so deeply ingrained that they form the foundation for the rest of your child's life. Likewise, if a child or adolescent does not learn to recognize and acknowledge emotions as normal and appropriate, the adult that child becomes will be likely to eat for emotional reasons.

Good for You!

By reading this book you have made the commitment, as a family, to confront the problems faced by your overweight child. Let me congratulate you! The positive changes you and your child are making will enhance all your lives.

Give yourself a big pat on the back. If you were one of our patients, everyone in our office would do that. We love success stories. Nothing makes us happier than to see a child with a weight problem turn her life around.

The six chapters you have read so far have probably kicked you off to a good start. I suspect that the appendix will rarely be far from your side. It contains a treasure of ideas, lists, goals—some of which you probably have mined already.

Before we leave you to the final chapter, we need to launch an unpleasant task. Until we all live in a perfect world, we have to face the reality that some families exhibit less than ideal relationships. As promised from time to time throughout the book, we will now look at extreme conditions that can influence a child's weight problem.

Eating Disorders—Warning Signs and What to Do

Our society puts too much pressure on children and adolescents to be pencil-thin. According to current U.S. statistics, about 60 percent of girls and 25 percent of boys in high school are on diets, even though 50 percent of these dieting high schoolers are either normal or underweight. Children do go to extremes, as they haven't gained the maturity to know when enough is enough. However, a significant number of children—particularly adolescents—fall into the quagmire of an eating disorder. In fact, eating disorders are the third most common chronic illness among adolescent girls, and one out of ten teens suffers from a clinical eating disorder.[1]

A recent Health Canada study found that both girls and boys between ten and sixteen struggle with perceptions of body image, with more than one third of all thirteen-year-old girls and nearly half of all fifteen-year-old girls feeling they need to lose weight.[2]

We won't get too technical about eating disorders, but it is important to define them so you can be on the look-out. *Anorexia* manifests as an intense fear of becoming obese. This fear does not diminish as weight decreases. The person suffering from this psychological illness demonstrates a disturbance of body image, seeing herself as fat even when she is emaciated.

Bulimia is defined as recurrent episodes of binge eating: the rapid consumption of huge amounts of food in a discrete period of time, typically less than two hours. Note: this is different from the type of emotional binge represented by the vignette that opened this chapter. Bulimia involves frequent, recurring episodes, often accompanied by self-induced vomiting or the use of laxatives.

One of the warning signs of an eating disorder is a preoccupation with dieting and weight loss. If your child talks about being fat when she really is not, if she displays a rapid weight loss or major fluctuations in body weight, recognize these as possible indicators.

If your child, overweight or normal, suddenly begins an *excessive* exercise program or displays symptoms of hyperactivity, that could be a sign. Talk with your child in a casual, nonthreatening atmosphere and ask why she has decided to become so active. It could be that she just went overboard when exercise was advised. But it could be that she is heading toward a full-blown eating disorder.

Some with an eating disorder eat next to nothing; they push food around their plate but actually consume very little. Many times, they eat only a few types of foods, especially those with very low calorie values, thus jeopardizing their overall nutrition. Others will take in immense quantities of food—they go on binges—then induce vomiting. Notice whether your child disappears after eating; she may be in the bathroom poking her finger down her throat to throw up the food before it can be digested. In addition to vomiting, she may also take laxatives to rush food through her digestive system. A child with an eating disorder might, therefore, suffer from diarrhea, constipation, bloating or frequent stomach aches.

This is serious. People can die from eating disorders!

Please heed these warning signals and alert your pediatrician or family physician to your suspicions before your child irreparably damages her health. Your health-care provider may refer you to a qualified eating disorder counselor, a psychologist or psychiatrist.

Could Abuse Be an Issue in Your Family?

Another condition that affects a child's weight is the presence of abuse in the family. Once taboo as topics of conversation, physical, emotional, and sexual abuse have been around for generations. Literature is filled with appalling stories of extreme forms of discipline that are nothing more than child-beating and verbal torture. Incest, once kept as the darkest of family secrets, has gouged its way out of the depths of denial. Today we acknowledge the existence of these abuses and recognize them as symbolic of dysfunctional family interaction. Finally, our society has taken steps to prosecute such abuse as criminal.

A child fighting the threat of physical, verbal, or sexual abuse often resorts to gaining weight as a form of protection. The child believes, sadly, that by being overweight, she will become less attractive to the abuser or, conversely, powerful enough to fend it off. The weight problem is merely a manifestation of these deeper, more serious, issues. (Although throughout the book we have used the feminine pronoun, please keep in mind that boys are also victims of these kinds of abuse.)

Make yourself aware of possibilities. Don't think that it couldn't happen in your household. These types of abuse know no barriers of economic or social status. Be aware of a change in your child's personality. Such abuse frequently causes the child to be severely depressed. If your child exhibits extreme stress when in the presence of a particular person, it could be a sign that abuse is happening when you're not around. The abuser need not be a member of the immediate family; it could be a more distant relative or even a neighbor or "friend."

Should you have suspicions, you need to consult a health-care professional. Start by detailing the signs you've noticed, in a frank talk with your family physician or pediatrician, who can refer you to appropriate counselors, and even to police if official intervention is required.

This is tough work, and you cannot be expected to tackle it on your own. These situations place a terrible burden on the entire family. But saving your child from lifelong debilitation is worth the effort.

May you possess the courage to face and conquer the problem.

Chapter Recap

* K.C. indulges in an episode of binge eating, a symptom of some emotional issues going on in her life. This is a good time for her parents to reinforce their unconditional love and help her learn better ways to deal with these emotions.

* Anger, boredom, anxiety, and fear can generate the urge to eat. Children with a weight problem need to learn to recognize and acknowledge these emotions and to substitute alternate activities for eating. One alternative: committing themselves in their goal journal to do something constructive instead of bingeing.

* To determine whether the hunger she feels is physical or emotional, your child can set a kitchen timer for three minutes. If she's still hungry at the "ding," she can go ahead and eat.

* Family and friends, even without realizing it, can sabotage a child's efforts to establish a healthier lifestyle. Role play various responses your child can give to family and friends when confronted with temptations. The occasional birthday cake or holiday treats won't undo all the good that's been done. More important than sticking with a diet is for your child not to feel left out of festivities with peers.

* Practice some words of wisdom to pass along to your child when she does have a relapse. Be prepared; it will happen.

* Prevention of lifelong obesity is definitely within your child's reach. Address it early rather than late—the earlier, the better.

* Congratulate yourself and your family for pursuing the commitment to help the overweight child you love. You and your entire family have earned a hearty "well done."

* Be alert to the signs of some serious issues that can affect a child's weight. Eating disorders can be fatal, so consult a professional if your child shows the signs of anorexia or bulimia. Likewise, do not ignore the possibility that your child is a victim of abuse; and, once again, consult a professional to help you tackle this serious situation.

Seven

K.C. Reaches Her Goals

"You really worried about me that much?" Alexa asked K.C. at school on Monday.

"Of course I'm worried about you. For the last two weeks you've been someone I don't even know. You don't talk. Every time I look at you, you're on the verge of crying. Your grades have tanked." K.C. plunked her backpack onto the table and pulled Alexa to a seat. "So what's up? You ready to spill it?"

Alexa squeezed K.C.'s hand. "I just can't get over that you ate all that junk because you were worried about me. You've been doing so great. Sara and I are so proud of you."

"Stop avoiding my question. Yeah, I went on a binge on Saturday, but it wasn't just you. Lots of other emotional stuff, too. I've already put it into my journal and cleared the air with my mom and dad. We're cool." K.C. looked into Alexa's eyes. "Now, before the bell rings, what's up? Are you okay?"

"If you call hating life 'okay,' then I'm okay." Alexa sighed then rushed on. "I didn't want to say anything till it was definite. We're moving away."

"What? You can't! . . . When? Where?"

"Mom got a big promotion and has to move to her company's home office in Boston. Dad will stay with us and continue his job here till the house sells. I hope it never sells!"

"Are they getting . . . ?"

"Divorced? No, they're real excited about moving to the city. Dad can find a job there, no sweat. They say we'll love it once we get over the hassle of moving. How can I love living so far from you and Sara? My life is ruined."

K.C. sat quietly, taking it all in. No wonder Alexa had acted so strange lately. She already felt a hole in her heart, even though it could be months before she'd have to say good-bye to her dear friend. "We'll just have to make the most of whatever time we have together," she said at last.

"K.C., let me say this now, because when it's time to move, I may not be able to."

"Yes? What is it?"

"You can't believe how proud I am of you, how glad I am to have you as my friend."

"Me, too."

"No, really, I've watched you change so much since this time last year. Look at you—you're happy. And gorgeous!"

K.C. grinned. "Get real. I'm not gorgeous, but I am comfortable with my size."

"You're never going to be thin, that's true. But that won't keep you from being awesome. Nobody—but nobody—teases you anymore."

"Yeah, not even my stupid brother."

"I know how hard it was for you, K.C.—your whole family, really. You've helped me, too, whether you know it or not."

"But you were never fat."

"No, but you taught me how to look at options, set goals, work toward them. Do you have any idea how important all that is? I do. My parents do. They're doing the same things right now, as they make plans for this big change in our lives. And we owe it all to you."

"I feel good about it myself. Dr. Cederquist says that I've made the kind of lifestyle changes that I can stick to the rest of my life, so I will be a healthy adult. And, believe it or not, I actually enjoy having exercise in my life now. It's done wonders for me. Not just helping me slim down but I actually feel better when I'm active. It's nice not having so much weight to drag around."

"You were always a smart kid, K.C., but now you have a plan for your whole life, goals that you didn't have before."

"Not for my *whole* life, you silly goose. I just turned twelve!"

"Get real. I've read some of your journal entries. Maybe the doctor taught you how to use those journals in her weight-management program, but you've taken them even further. No matter what kind of problem you ever face in your life, you can handle it because you've learned how to handle anything."

"I never thought of it like that." K.C. stood up just as the bell sounded. "I wasn't happy when I was twenty pounds overweight last year, but I guess I can be thankful that being that heavy made me learn how to change my life." K.C. hugged Alexa to her. "C'mon, grab your books and let's get to first period."

Appendix

Appendix One

Journals

Not only has our K.C. recovered from her emotion-inspired binge, she has dealt with it in a positive manner by writing about it in her journal. In fact, her journals have become a significant factor in her life. They help her to analyze options, set goals, and assess progress toward achieving them.

Let's take a closer look at the concept of keeping journals and how your K.C. can benefit from them in her own life.

Help Your Child to Organize Three Journals

Some people find a journal easier to organize if it covers only one topic. If your K.C. is like that, buy her three separate notebooks. Get the loose-leaf kind so that she can easily add and subtract pages. If each one is a different color, she can tell at a glance which one to grab for that moment's task. The "Eating" journal might be green, the color associated with healthy vegetables. You might choose red for the "Exercise" journal, to remind her that she needs to exercise long enough to get her heart rate up and some color into her cheeks. For "Emotions," blue would be a serene, comforting color.

Others like to keep all their notations in one loose-leaf notebook with tabs to mark the three sections. If your K.C. prefers one to three, get her a notebook that can be decorated with stickers, paints, or colored pens. Suggest that she doodle on the outside as she thinks about what she will write on the inside. If she's making an entry about food, her doodle could be an apple or a head of broccoli—something to remind her of healthy eating. For exercise, she could draw a symbol suggestive of movement—an arrow, for example. A "smiley face" might encourage her to write about her emotions. Allow her to be as creative as she wants. It is *her* journal, not to be read by anyone else unless she so chooses.

Private or Shared? Your Child's Choice

In the vignette in chapter 7, Alexa refers to K.C.'s journal. Obviously, K.C. shared some of it with her friends. Sharing with close friends is normal but not absolutely necessary. Let your child decide whether to keep it totally private or let those close to her know what's in it.

When members of my staff and I work with patients, we ask them to make several commitments to the program. One of them is to keep just the kinds of journals that I'm describing. To make certain they are keeping their end of the deal, we ask to see the journals—not to read the entries, but merely to leaf through and see that there are notations in every section, or in every type of journal if they keep separate ones. Once the patients realize that we will occasionally check on them, they become more diligent in making entries. Then, in a few weeks, after trust has been established and they have begun to comprehend for themselves the benefits of journal keeping, we merely ask them how their journals are coming but don't leaf through them. You can follow the same process in your home.

On the other hand, some patients use journal entries to trigger discussion with me, our nutritionist or our exercise physiologist. I've had them read aloud one of their entries, then we talk about the questions it raised. Again, you can do the same thing at home.

Remember, earlier in this book, I suggested that you establish an atmosphere of open communication with your child, especially as to her feelings about her weight. Once she starts writing about her feelings in the journal, you can ask her if she'd like to share any of the entries with you. A child frequently feels things she has trouble expressing. She doesn't know if she's "normal" in feeling as she does, so you can help her understand that everyone goes through the same kinds of emotions as they grow up. By helping her acknowledge and deal with her emotions, you may build the foundation of a lifelong closeness between parent and child.

How to Journal

Now, let's get down to business on how to journal. Some people merely jot down key words at the time they experience a problem and flesh out the entry later. Others schedule a journal time as part of their daily routine—most often just before going to bed—and review the day on the "movie screen" in their mind. They pick out anything significant and write about it as fully or as simply as suits their own personal style.

The "Eating" Journal

We in our office feel that our patients benefit greatly if they start their Eating journal by writing down every bite that goes into their mouths for the first four weeks of their weight-management program. Some continue to do this all the time. It often turns out to be a real eye-opener.

Typically, overweight people have no idea how much they eat or what they eat. Once they take "Nutrition 101" (chapter 3), some realize that it's not entirely *how much* they eat but that they have become used to eating the *wrong* things. So, Rule Number One is for your K.C. to keep track of *everything* that goes into her mouth for the first few weeks. Yes, even chewing gum.

Each entry should be dated, e.g., August 20, Sunday. Breakfast . . . Lunch . . . Dinner . . . Snacks (mid-morning, mid-afternoon, evening, whatever is the case). Describe the portion sizes in a meaningful way. For example, a serving of macaroni and cheese might be the size of a fist or the size of a plum. Your K.C. can choose words that mean something to her. Explain any special circumstance, such as a birthday party, an episode of binge eating, etc. Be sure to reference any unusual eating in the Emotions journal, as there will probably be a connection.

Over the weeks, as your K.C. changes her diet to substitute healthier foods for those high in fat or sugar, she is sure to notice a difference in the kinds of foods she consumes. In addition, portion sizes will grow smaller; empty calories will be eliminated or greatly reduced. Success builds on success, so as she approaches her goals, she will probably journal fewer binges, less appetite for junk food.

The "Exercise" Journal

Your child's Exercise journal can follow the same format. Start with the date, then write down *every activity* that involves moving. Yes, that includes walking from the car parked at the back of the lot to the mall entrance. She'll be trying different kinds of exercise to find her favorites. Again, as she makes each effort, she can reference how she feels about it in the Emotions journal. In this way, she can decide whether to stick with in-line skating over walking or swimming instead of jogging. All provide exercise, but if she *likes* one better than another, she will be more likely to continue doing it.

The same goes with organized sports. Through trial and error, your child may develop an untapped prowess at soccer, tennis, or golf. Once she discovers where her natural talents lie, she will get more enjoyment out of exercising in that sport. It will become a mainstay of her life, throughout childhood and into adulthood. She can follow her own development by reviewing the daily notes in her Exercise journal.

Once your child has altered her eating and exercise habits to the healthy ones she will follow for the rest of her life, these two journals will become less important and may even be set aside. However, the Emotions journal is different. Many people keep this kind of journal forever.

The "Emotions" Journal

To make the Emotions journal really work, help your child to understand that feelings are normal and not to be ignored or explained away as a "silly" reaction. In her journal, she can learn to get to the bottom of what she is really feeling, even if the surface emotion seems to be a different one. Do you recall how we talked about fear lying beneath anger? That's what I mean. A journal entry often leads a person to discover what is really going on in her emotional world.

Everyone has fears. Children and adolescents have fears squared! They see a complicated, sometimes brutal, world and wonder how they will fit into it. What will they *be* when they grow up? (Adults feed this fear by asking repeated questions before the child has any idea where her abilities might lead her.) In some areas of high crime, sorry to say, children even wonder if they *will* grow up.

Is popularity within their reach? Will they wear the right clothes, follow the current styles in makeup, hair? Will they have lots of friends? Will they flunk chemistry? Can their parents afford to send them to college? Will they get married or stay single? Will their marriage be a happy one or miserable? Will they make lots of money or live at the edge of poverty? In short, they tend to worry about everything, and worry is born of fear.

Writing in the Emotions journal offers an outlet for fears that might otherwise be fed by overeating. When a child suffers a crushing emotional blow followed by a relapse to old eating habits, writing about the relapse in the journal helps the child to analyze what happened and why. Understanding the process of emotional overeating can help to eliminate it. That "aha!" experience becomes liberating and the child, now aware, is freed from the emotional prison built on ignorance of why she did something.

The Importance of Goals

Let me suggest that all three of the journals work better if they include goals. These goals can be either self-imposed or agreed upon with other members of the family. They offer a progress chart that documents how well your child is doing in each significant area of lifestyle growth or change.

In our office, we find that some people have never attempted to define possible goals, decide which ones to pursue, and chart their progress toward attainment. If that is the case in your household, don't worry. It is not a formidable task but quite easy once you realize that you are in control at all points in the process.

Let's work with one example already alluded to in chapter 6. You'll recall that I mentioned a patient who, when she had some kind of emotional crisis, cleaned her closet or dresser drawers instead of eating. Here's how she might have arrived at that decision in her Emotions journal.

Definition of goal: to substitute productive activity for emotional eating.

Possible activities:

1) bang head against wall—damaging to self and wall so *not* productive

2) beat up on kid brother— satisfying but would result in punishment

3) get out of house, away from temptation—not always possible

4) clean basement—do that only for money

5) rearrange dresser drawers—would help me find stuff faster

6) clean out closet, give old stuff to Goodwill—would make me feel charitable

7) clean and tidy room—parents would drop dead so *NOT* productive

By the process of evaluating each option she came up with, this person decided that numbers 5 and 6 made the most sense. Notice that she also tried to engage her sense of humor while thinking up and assessing each option.

Step One: Define the Goal

The first step for your K.C.—with your help, if she's too young to do it alone— is to define the goal she wants to establish. It may take several stabs before the goal is sufficiently refined to be reached. It should entail only one element. Not "try out for cheerleader so I'll be one of the most popular girls in school" but "try out for cheerleader." Is that the real goal? Or is it "make my body flexible enough to do the splits"? That's what I mean by a goal that is sufficiently refined. In this way, each major goal may be broken down into smaller ones that lead up to the main one.

Establish a Time Limit

Once a goal has been defined, then your child can establish a time for goal attainment. She has to be realistic. She won't be doing the splits in one week, unless her body already has a large degree of flexibility. She might give herself six months then be super pleased with herself if she reaches the goal in half that time!

Chart Progress toward Lifestyle Changes

Encourage your child to come up with goals that will help her make the lifestyle changes necessary to conquer her weight problems. May I suggest *"Healthier Eating Goals," "Exercise Goals,"* and *"Emotional Goals."* These could be placed on the first sheet of paper in each journal, so that she can review them every time she opens the notebook.

Take a step-by-step approach to make the goal a stretch but reachable. For example, in the first week of the program, if your K.C. adores sweets, her Healthier Eating goal might be to have only two high-calorie desserts, like cake or pie, during that week. For someone used to eating a sweet every day, that goal will require self-discipline, but it is definitely attainable. If reducing it to *two* seems unreasonable in the first week, set *three* or *four* as the goal. What we want is progress toward the goal of *one*. If the reduction goes from seven to one in the first week, the frustration of doing without may sabotage the effort.

If junk food is your K.C.'s primary snack, one of her Healthier Eating goals will be to substitute a healthier snack, such as fresh fruit or unbuttered popcorn. Once again, a gradual reduction is more likely to be successful. Start with substitutions four days a week, then five, six, then eventually every day.

Mark successful progress in some way. A simple plus sign might say "Hooray," while a minus sign says "Not today." A quick glance at pluses and minuses can make your child feel good about her progress.

Sample Goal Page from "Eating" Journal

At the end of the week, the first page of the Eating journal might wind up looking something like this:

GOAL	SUN	MON	TUE	WED	THU	FRI	SAT	MET
Week beginning September 10:								
Fruit for mid-morning snack 3X	+	-	-	+	-	-	+	☺
Veggie for after-school snack 4X	-	+	+	+	+	-	-	☺
No cakes, cookies, candy 2X	-	-	+	-	+	-	-	☺
Do not clean plate at dinner 5X	+	-	+	-	-	+	+	
Drink water instead of soda 6X	+	+	+	+	+	+	-	☺

Eventual goal: do all every day by end of fourth week

GOAL	SUN	MON	TUE	WED	THU	FRI	SAT	MET
Week beginning September 17:								
Fruit for mid-morning snack 4X	+	-	+	-	-	-*	+	
Veggie for after-school snack 5X	-	+	+	+	+	+	-	☺
No cakes, cookies, candy 5X	-	-	+	+	+	-	-	
Do not clean plate at dinner 7X	+	+	+	-	+	+	+	
Drink water instead of soda 7X	+	+	+	+	+	+	+	☺
Eat healthy breakfast 7X	+	+	+	+	-*	+	-*	

GOAL	SUN	MON	TUE	WED	THU	FRI	SAT	MET
Week beginning September 24:								
Fruit for mid-morning snack 4X	+	-	+	+	-	-	+	☺
Veggie for late afternoon snack 7X	+	+	+	+	+	+	+	☺
No cakes, pies, candy 7X	-	+	+	+	+	+	-*	
Do not clean plate at dinner 7X	+	+	+	-	+	+	+	
Drink water instead of soda 7X	+	+	+	+	+	+	+	☺
Eat healthy breakfast 7X	+	+	+	+	-*	+	-*	
Cut portion sizes by 1/4 7X	+	+	+	+	+	+	+	☺

Eventual goal: cut portion sizes by 1/2 by end of fourth week

Sometimes the goals will be met, sometimes they won't. Maybe they were a little unreasonable, and the next week will be better. The significant factor is the awareness that journaling creates. They make goals concrete and visual—something specific to work on.

Note the asterisks? They indicate that there will be a reference to this in the Emotions journal. When the goal isn't reached on that day, it is good to explain what happened. Your K.C. might oversleep one morning and be too late to eat a healthy breakfast so she grabs something quick—a doughnut, perhaps. A minus sign for that day won't explain the reason for not making the goal, but an entry in the Emotions journal will.

When your K.C. attains a goal she has set for herself that week, she needs to mark it in some way.

Buy some congratulatory stickers, available in supply stores for teachers and, possibly, in your local department store. I've seen some that say "Way to go!" "Attagirl!" "Attaboy!" "Congratulations!" "You Did It!" Others are smiley faces in various sizes. Tell your child you have them and what you want her to do with them. When your K.C. asks for a sticker to place in her journal, you'll know she's done something worthy of a reward. Praise her! Maybe she'll even tell you what it is, tightening the bond between parent and child.

Become Aware of Patterns

Patterns may also become apparent. Notice in our example that sweets seem to show up every Saturday. Why? What is different about that day? Because it's not a school day and routines are relaxed? Because that's time spent with friends, when temptations are high? Because from long habit, the family enjoys sweet desserts on Saturday? Goes out for pancakes or waffles for breakfast? Visits Grandma?

At first, when it is harder for your child to get away from old habits and into healthier ones, suggest that it's better if the "off" days for such goals coincide with special family occasions. Later, once the new habits are well established, your child will be better able to resist temptations on those days and pulses will replace most minus signs.

Also note that each week builds on the week before. Start with the goals already established for the previous week, whether they were successfully met or not. Increase the number of times or leave them the same, depending on what is potentially attainable for the week coming up. For example, if your child knows she will attend a birthday party this week, she will take that into consideration when setting how many days she will not have sweets. Then add a new goal. Your child may be surprised at how quickly all the minuses disappear from the chart!

Sample Goal Page from "Exercise" Journal

Follow the same format for the Exercise goals. The first page in that journal might look like this:

GOAL	SUN	MON	TUE	WED	THU	FRI	SAT	MET
Week beginning September 10:								
Walk one mile 4X	+	-	+	+	-	-	+	☺
Take tennis lessons at Y 2X	-	-	-	+	-	-	+	☺

Eventual goal: increase walk to two miles by end of third week, to three miles by end of sixth.

GOAL	SUN	MON	TUE	WED	THU	FRI	SAT	MET
Week beginning September 17:								
Walk one mile 4X	+	-	+	+	-	-	+	☺
Take tennis lessons at Y 2X	-	-	-	+	-	-	+	☺
Swim one hour after tennis 1X	-	-	-	-	-	-	+	☺

GOAL	SUN	MON	TUE	WED	THU	FRI	SAT	MET
Week beginning September 24:								
Walk one mile 5X	+	-	+	-	+	+	+	☺
Take tennis lessons at Y 2X	-	-	-	+	-	-	+	☺
Swim one hour after tennis 2X	-	-	-	+	-	-	+	☺
Jump rope for 5 minutes 3X	-	-*	-	+	-	-	+	

This sample chart merits a smiley face, don't you think? Only one asterisk, and that next to what might have been the first day set to try this new goal. Walking for one mile four or five days a week seems to fit well into this person's schedule. It won't be too difficult to extend that to every day! As the weight starts to come down, she will be able to walk at a faster pace and push for two miles, then three in the same time it first took her to walk one mile!

Swimming for an hour after tennis went from once to twice in one week. Our sample person *likes* this exercise. She'll probably build on that enjoyment in later goals. Jumping rope, a pretty intense exercise, needs some work. Maybe next week she should cut her goal down to twice. Or maybe three times but only three minutes each time. If she wrote about it in her Emotions journal, as the asterisk indicates, she will be able to determine how to reassess that goal.

Sample Goal Page from "Emotions" Journal

Setting goals at the beginning of the Emotions journal might take a different format, similar to the example used earlier: to replace emotional eating with a productive activity. These goals will grow out of your child's actual experiences. If anger or crying is an everyday occurrence, then it would be appropriate to follow the same format used in the other two journals, to reduce and eventually eliminate the negative emotional outbursts. (For example, "won't cry when teased" four days first week, five the second, seven by end of fourth week.) However, most of the time your child will be dealing with situational emotions and, therefore, will be hard-pressed to establish goals until the situation that elicits the emotion actually occurs.

Let's look at another example of defining a goal in the Emotions journal and assessing options that will help achieve it.

Definition of goal: to react to teasing about my weight without crying or getting mad.

Options:

1) Tease the teaser right back—could result in a bloody nose, possibly mine

2) Rehearse snappy comebacks—might take too long to decide which one to use

3) Say "Sticks and stones may break my bones but words will never hurt me."—would have to act like I believe it

4) Shut out the teasers by opening a book, gazing out the window, talking to a friend, closing my eyes and thinking about a beautiful place—if they realize they aren't getting to me, they'll quit. I choose option # 4.

Just as in the other journals, it is important to note progress in some way. Have your child write down the date on which a situation occurs that leads to a new Emotions goal. Then, the next time the same situation comes up and she responds in the way she chose, she can reward herself.

Appendix Two

Primary Goal: Healthier Lifestyle Habits

As promised throughout this book, we have included various lists of healthier selections that can help your child reach her primary goal: to establish healthier habits she can follow for the rest of her life. We placed these lists at the end of the book so that you could quickly turn to them when the occasion arose. We wouldn't be surprised if they comprise what will become the most-thumbed section of the book.

Let me emphasize what we have said several times in various ways: we don't want to take away all the goodies from an overweight child. Life without the enjoyment of an occasional piece of cake, pizza, or candy bar would be no fun. We have no intention of insisting that success is out of reach if your child ever steps foot in a fast-food restaurant. Dining out—even in a fast-food place—is now and will long remain a fact of life in our society. At home, there's breakfast, and then there's a healthier breakfast. And lunch. And dinner. And snack. These lists will help make those healthier choices that will get your child to her goals.

Healthier Choices in Fast Food

Not all the foods we will list do we consider "healthy." What we try to do here is show you how to make "healthier" choices from some that offer incredibly high levels of fat or sugar or calories. Please understand that we make no attempt to be comprehensive. When you eat at one of these fast-food restaurants, just be aware of ways to limit your intake of the less desirable nutrients.

Index Reference

Cal   Calories
Fat   Fat (grams)
%Fc   Percent of Calories from Fat
S. Fat   Saturated Fat (grams)
Sod   Sodium (milligrams)

Restaurants

Arby's

Food Name	Calories	Fat	S. Fat	% Fc	Sodium
Better Choice					
Garden Salad	60	1	0	7	40
Roast Beef Deluxe	295	10	3	31	825
Roast Chicken Deluxe	275	6	2	23	775
Roast Turkey Deluxe	260	7	2	21	1260
Roast Chicken Deluxe	150	2	1	12	420
Side Salad	25	0	0	12	15
Baked Potato - Plain	355	0	0	0	25
As Compared To					
Sandwiches					
Beef 'N Cheddar	490	28	9	52	1215
Junior Roast Beef	325	14	5	39	780
Regular Roast Beef	390	19	7	44	1010
Super Roast Beef	525	27	9	46	1190
Chicken Cordon Blue	625	33	8	48	1595
Grilled Chicken Deluxe	430	20	4	42	850

Food Name	Calories	Fat	S. Fat	% Fc	Sodium
Roast Chicken Club	545	31	9	51	1105
Curly Fries	300	15	3	45	855
Cheddar Curly Fries	335	18	4	48	1015

Tips

Some selections at this fast-food place don't look so bad in the calorie and fat categories, but do be watchful of the sodium amounts if you need to restrict that nutrient.

Boston Market

Food Name	Calories	Fat	S. Fat	% Fc	Sodium
Better Choice					
Chicken, 1/4 White Meat, w/o skin	160	4	1	20	350
Chicken, 1/4 Dark Meat, w/o skin	210	10	3	43	320
Turkey Breast, w/o skin	170	1	1	5	850
Chicken Soup (3/4 Cup)	80	3	1	34	470
Sandwiches (no cheese or sauce):					
Chicken	430	5	1	10	910
Ham	450	9	3	18	1600
Ham & Turkey Club	460	6	2	13	1330
Turkey	400	4	1	8	1070
Corn (3/4 Cup)	190	4	1	19	130
Rice Pilaf (2/3 Cup)	180	5	1	25	600
As Compared To					
Chicken, 1/4 White Meat w/skin	330	17	5	46	530
Chicken, 1/4 Dark Meat w/skin	330	22	6	60	460
Chicken Tortilla Soup (1 Cup)	220	11	4	45	1410
Caesar Salad Entree (10 oz.)	520	43	12	74	1420
Tortellini Salad (3/4 Cup)	380	24	5	57	530
Sandwiches (with cheese and sauce):					
Chicken	750	33	12	38	1860
Ham	760	35	13	41	1880
Ham & Turkey Club	890	44	20	43	2350
Turkey	710	28	10	35	1390
Coleslaw (3/4 Cup)	280	16	3	51	520
Macaroni Cheese (3/4 Cup)	280	10	6	32	760

Tips

Always order chicken without skin or remove it before you eat it. Also, say no to the cheese and sauces.

Burger King

Food Name	Calories	Fat	S. Fat	% Fc	Sodium
Better Choice					
Whopper Jr. Sandwich w/o Mayo	320	15	7	44	460
Hamburger	320	15	6	42	530
Bk Broiler Chicken Sandwich w/o Mayo	370	9	4	22	90
Barbecue - Dipping Sauce	35	0	0	0	40
Honey Flavored - Dipping Sauce	90	0	0	0	10
Sweet & Sour - Dipping Sauce	45	0	0	0	50
As Compared To					
Whopper Sandwich	660	40	12	54	900
Whopper Jr. Sandwich	400	24	8	54	530
Bacon Double Cheeseburger	620	38	18	55	1230
Bk Big Fish Sandwich	720	43	9	54	1180
Bk Broiler Chicken Sandwich	530	26	5	43	1060
French Fries, Medium	400	21	8	47	820
French Fries, Large	590	30	12	46	1180
Onion Rings, Medium	380	19	2	45	550
Ranch - Dipping Sauce	170	17	3	90	200

Tips

Notice that two sandwiches appear in both lists. What makes one a "better" choice? *No mayo!* Look at those fat calories— nearly all above the recommended 30 percent. Only the BK Broiler Chicken Sandwich— hold the mayo— falls under that point. If you must have a dipping sauce, choose one that *isn't* Ranch!

Chick-Fil-A

Food Name	Calories	Fat	S. Fat	% Fc	Sodium
Better Choice					
Sandwiches:					
Chicken	290	9	2	27	870
Chicken Deluxe	300	9	2	27	870
Chargrilled Chicken	280	3	1	11	640
Chargrilled Deluxe Chicken	290	3	1	10	640
Chicken Salad On Whole Wheat	320	5	2	12	810
Hearty Breast of Chicken Soup	110	1	0	8	760
Chargrilled Chicken Garden Salad	170	3	1	18	650
Chicken Salad Plate	290	5	0	14	570
Carrot & Raisin Salad, Small	150	2	0	13	650
As Compared To					
Chicken Nuggets, 8-Pack	290	14	3	52	770
Waffle Potato Fries	290	10	4	31	960

Food Name	Calories	Fat	S. Fat	% Fc	Sodium
Lemon Pie, Slice	280	22	6	71	550
Cheesecake with Topping	290	23	10	72	550

Tip

These values look pretty good, especially when compared to some of the other fast-food restaurants. Just stay away from the desserts, whose calories from fat soar way beyond the desired 30 percent.

Dairy Queen / Brazier

Food Name	Calories	Fat	S. Fat	% Fc	Sodium
Better Choice					
Grilled Chicken Sandwich w/o Cheese	310	10	3	29	1040
DQ Vanilla Soft Serve, 1/2 Cup	140	4	3	26	70
DQ Choc. Soft Serve, 1/2 Cup	150	5	4	30	75
Cup of Frozen Yogurt, Regular	230	1	0	2	150
As Compared To					
Bacon Double Cheeseburger	610	36	18	53	1380
Chili 'N Cheese Dog	330	21	9	57	1090
Chicken Breast Fillet Sandwich	430	20	4	42	760
Grilled Chicken Sandwich w/Cheese	480	25	7	47	980
Buster Bar	450	28	12	56	280
Choc. Chip Cookie Dough Blizzard, Reg.	950	36	19	34	660
Dilly Bar, Chocolate	210	13	7	56	75
Heath Breeze (Yogurt), Regular	710	18	11	23	580

Tip

If you have to order something at Dairy Queen other than the Soft Serve, stick with the grilled chicken.

Denny's

Food Name	Calories	Fat	S. Fat	% Fc	Sodium
Better Choice					
Hot Cakes, Plain	490	7	1	13	1820
Ham, 3 oz.	95	3	1	28	760
English Muffin, Each	125	1	0	7	20
Oatmeal, 4 oz.	100	2	0	18	175
Chicken Noodle Soup	60	2	0	30	640
Split Pea Soup	145	6	2	37	820
Garden Chick. Delite Salad, No Dress.	277	5	1	16	785
Side Garden Salad	115	4	1	31	150
French Dip w/ Horseradish Sandwich	530	16	3	39	1895
Grilled Chicken Sandwich	510	20	5	35	1810
Grilled Chicken Dinner	130	4	1	28	560

As Compared To

Food Name	Calories	Fat	S. Fat	% Fc	Sodium
American Slam w/Biscuit	1405	109	26	70	2675
Original Grand Slam w/Syrup & Marg.	1030	60	16	52	2385
Scram Slam w/1 Slice Toast	1065	81	23	68	1915
Ham 'n Cheddar Omelet	745	55	10	66	1520
Chicken Fried Steak and Eggs	725	55	18	68	1505
Steak and Eggs (Porterhouse)	1225	95	32	68	1370
Waffles, Plain	305	21	3	63	200
Waffles, w/Syrup And Butter	540	31	5	52	345
Hot Cakes w/Syrup and Butter	725	17	3	21	1965
Biscuit w/Sausage and Gravy	570	38	10	60	1475
Cream of Broccoli Soup	195	12	9	55	820
Cream of Potato Soup	220	12	9	49	760
Buffalo Chicken Salad, No Dressing	615	37	8	54	1260
Fried Chicken Salad, No Dressing	505	31	8	55	1175
Classic Burger	675	40	15	53	1140
Deluxe Grilled Cheese	480	26	2	49	1135
Fisherman's Choice	905	56	8	55	1705
Buffalo Wings (12)	855	54	17	57	5550
Burgerlicious w/Cheese-Kids Meal	340	20	6	53	580
The Big Cheese-Kids Meal	334	20	2	54	830
Dennysaur Chicken Nuggets-Kids Meal	190	13	4	61	340

Tips

Get a load of the sodium in those buffalo wings! In fact, quite a few of the menu selections at this restaurant rank higher than I like in the sodium category. But if sodium is not a problem, be sure to select according to the values for calories from fat, as I'm sure you have learned by now.

Kentucky Fried Chicken

Food Name	Calories	Fat	S. Fat	% Fc	Sodium
Better Choice					
Tender Roast, no skin	170	5	1	21	800
BBQ Flavored Chicken Sandwich	255	8	1	28	780
BBQ Baked Beans	190	3	1	14	760
Corn on the Cob	150	2	1	14	20
As Compared To					
Chicken Breast - Original Recipe	400	24	6	54	1120
Chicken Breast - Extra Crispy	470	28	7	54	930
Chicken Breast - Hot & Spicy	530	35	8	58	1110
Chunky Chicken Pot Pie	770	42	13	49	2160

Tip

Because the Original Recipe, Extra Crispy, and Hot & Spicy varieties are fried, by far your better choice is the Tender Roast without the skin. These values should be *big* eye-openers!

McDonald's

Food Name	Calories	Fat	S. Fat	% Fc	Sodium
Better Choice					
Grilled Chicken Deluxe, no Mayo	300	5	1	15	930
Hamburger	270	10	4	33	580
Cheeseburger	320	14	6	37	770
French fries, Small	210	10	2	43	135
Grilled Chicken Salad Deluxe	120	2	0	11	240
Garden Salad	35	0	0	0	20
Fat-Free Herb Vinaigrette, 1 pkg.	50	0	0	0	330
Egg McMuffin	290	12	5	37	710
Low-fat Apple Bran Muffin	300	3	1	90	380
Vanillla Reduced-Fat Ice Cream Cone	150	5	3	27	75
As Compared To					
Big Mac	560	31	10	50	1110
Fish Filet Deluxe	560	28	6	45	1060
Crispy Chicken Deluxe	500	25	4	45	1100
French fries, Super Size	540	26	5	43	350
Chicken McNugget, 6 Pieces	290	17	4	53	510
Ranch Salad Dressing, 1 Pkg.	230	21	3	82	550
Caesar Salad Dressing, 1 Pkg.	160	14	3	79	450
Sausage McMuffin w/egg	440	28	10	57	810
Bacon, Egg & Cheese Biscuit	440	26	8	52	1300
Baked Apple Pie	260	13	4	45	00

Tips

You *can* eat at McDonald's and not blow it, but it isn't easy. Watch for the percentage of calories from fat and select something that is under the 30 percent maximum we want in the daily diet. Ask them to leave off the mayo or special sauce. If you get a sandwich high in calories, then don't get fries or dessert. If you choose a salad, then you can top off your lunch with an ice cream cone.

Subway

Cheese and condiments not included; values for the 6" sub:

Food Name	Calories	Fat	S. Fat	% Fc	Sodium
Better Choice					
Ham	300	5	1	15	1320
Roast Beef	305	5	2	15	940
Subway Club	310	5	2	15	1350
Turkey Breast	290	4	1	12	1405
Turkey & Ham	295	5	2	15	1360
Veggie Delite	240	3	1	11	590
Roasted Chicken Breast	350	6	2	15	980
Ham Deli Style Sandwich	235	4	2	15	775

Caroline J. Cederquist, M.D.

Food Name	Calories	Fat	S. Fat	% Fc	Sodium
Roast Beef Deli Style Sandwich	245	4	1	15	640
Turkey Breast Deli Style Sandwich	235	4	1	15	945
Ham Salad	115	3	1	23	1035
Turkey Breast Salad	100	2	1	18	1120
Veggie Delite Salad	50	1	0	20	310
Fat-Free Italian Salad Dressing, 1 Pkg.	20	0	0	0	610
Fat-Free French Salad Dressing, 1 Pkg.	70	0	0	0	390
As Compared To					
Classic Italian BMT	460	22	6	43	1665
Cold Cut Trio	380	13	4	31	1410
Tuna, Light Mayo	390	15	4	35	940
Pizza Sub w/Cheese	465	22	9	43	1620
Steak & Cheese	400	10	6	22	1115
Bologna Deli Style Sandwich	290	12	4	37	745
Classic Italian BMT Salad	275	20	8	65	1380
Creamy Italian Salad Dressing, 1 Pkg.	260	28	6	96	530
French Salad Dressing, 1 Pkg.	280	24	2	77	400
Thousand Island Salad Dressing, 1 Pkg.	260	28	0	96	620
Ranch Salad Dressing, 1 Pkg.	350	40	0	100	470

Tip
The "better" choices here offer you some fairly decent values in terms of calories, fat, and percentage of calories from fat. Watch the sodium, however.

Taco Bell

Food Name	Calories	Fat	S. Fat	% Fc	Sodium
Better Choice					
Soft Taco, Steak	200	7	3	32	500
Soft Taco, Light Chicken	180	5	1	25	660
Kid's Chicken Soft Taco	180	5	2	25	590
Chicken Burrito, Light	310	8	2	21	980
As Compared To					
Taco, Regular	170	10	4	53	280
Soft Taco, Regular	210	10	5	43	530
Soft Taco, BLT	340	23	8	60	610
Kids's Soft Taco Roll-Up	280	15	8	48	790
Mexican Pizza	570	36	11	57	1050
Nachos, Big Beef Nachos Supreme	430	24	7	50	720
Nachos, BellGrande	740	39	10	47	1200

Tip
The chart values speak for themselves. If your friends insist on going to Taco Bell, your best bets in terms of percentage of calories from fat, would be the light chicken soft tacos, both adult and kid's size.

Wendy's

Food Name	Calories	Fat	S. Fat	% Fc	Sodium
Better Choice					
Plain Single	360	16	6	40	580
Jr. Cheeseburger	320	13	6	37	830
Kids Meal - Hamburger	370	10	3	33	610
Kids Meal - Cheeseburger	320	13	6	37	830
Grilled Chicken	310	8	2	23	780
Fresh Stuffed Pita-Caesar/Gdn./Chick.	490	18	5	33	1320
Fresh Stuffed Pita - Garden Veggie	400	17	4	38	760
Side Salad	60	3	1	45	180
Barbeque Sauce, 1 Package	50	0	0	0	100
Wine Vinegar Dressing, 2 Tbs.	0	0	0	0	0
Baked Potato, Plain	310	0	0	0	25
Baked Potato, Sour Cream & Chives	380	6	4	14	40
Chili, Small	210	7	3	30	800
As Compared To					
Big Bacon Classic	580	30	12	46	1460
Blue Cheese Dressing, 2 Tbs.	180	19	3	100	180
Italian Caesar Dressing, 2 Tbs.	150	16	2	96	240
Baked Potato, Bacon & Cheese	530	18	4	30	1390
Baked Potato, Broccoli & Cheese	470	14	3	27	470
Baked Potato, Cheese	570	23	8	36	640
Baked Potato, Chili & Cheese	630	24	9	35	770
Chicken Nuggets, 5 Piece	230	16	3	63	470

Tips

When you see the difference in values when you have your baked potato plain as compared to anyway else, you get a good idea of how detrimental all those toppings really are. Also notice that the blue cheese dressing is 100% fat. Choose *anything* but that! A Jr. Cheeseburger and a side salad with wine vinegar dressing provide the same amount of fat as a baked potato with sour cream and chives but far higher percentage of calories from fat. I just want you to be aware!

Other Healthier Choices

If your family loves Chinese food, here's what to keep in mind when dining at one of your favorite restaurants. Much of this food is loaded with sodium, with the healthier choices being the egg roll (under 500 mg. each), hot and sour soup (under 2,000 mg. per cup) and stir-fried vegetables (just over 2,000 for a 4-cup serving). These also top the list for low-fat content and calories per the size serving noted above. The egg roll carries under 200 calories and about 11 grams of fat; the hot and sour at 115 and 5, and the veggies at 750 calories and 20 grams of fat. Go easy on the soy sauce if you need to watch your sodium intake, as it is loaded—over 1000 mg. per tablespoon. Choose steamed over fried rice and limit your serving to one cup. Dishes containing nuts, such as Kung Pao Chicken, often are very high in fat—

because of those nuts. High amounts of fat come from the oils used for cooking, and for high cholesterol levels, you can blame eggs used in the recipes for some dishes, such as Moo Shu.

Appendix Three

Healthier Choices When Dining At Home

We have included quite a few lists to help you make healthier choices of foods for the family to enjoy when dining at home. All the lists below contain items and/or brands that my staff or I have researched. Some brands are regional and may not be available in your part of the country.

My primary concern is in the amount of fat and, in some foods, sugar. I include sodium values in case your child's personal physician advises limiting sodium in the diet. Fat, sat(urated) fat and sugar are shown in grams; sodium in milligrams. Remember that your daily intake of fat should be limited to less than 30 percent of your total calories, so always look at the percentage of fat calories where available. *Please note*: When I show the number of grams of nutrients immediately following the food item, those figures indicate the criteria for the brands listed under the "better choice" heading.

Abbreviation Reference

Cal	Calories
Fat	Fat (grams)
Fiber	Fiber
Sugar	Sugar
%Fc	Percent of Calories from Fat
S. Fat	Saturated Fat (grams)
Sod	Sodium (milligrams)
F/F	Fat-free

Page References for Dining at Home Foods

Cereals

Serving size is approximately 1 oz.

Better choices contain < 7 grams of sugar per serving and < 3 grams of fat. This nation leads the world in choices of prepared cereals. The next time you shop for groceries, just take a really long look at the cereal aisle. Amazing, isn't it? So that our research can be as helpful to you as possible, we have included probably way more about cereals than you'll ever want to know. Can't fault us for not being thorough, right?

Food Name	Calories	Fat	Fiber	Sugar
Better Choice				
Nabisco Shredded Wheat Spoon Size	104	0	3	0
Kellogg's All Bran With Extra Fiber	50	1	15	0
General Mills Fiber One	60	1	13	0
Quaker Oats Puffed Rice	107	0	0	0
Nabisco Shredded Wheat 'N Bran	102	1	4	0
Quaker Oats Puffed Wheat	100	0	2	0
Quaker Oats Shredded Wheat	105	1	3	0
Quaker Oats Oat Bran	113	2	5	1
General Mills Cheerios	110	2	3	1
General Mills Rice Chex	116	0	1	2
General Mills Country Corn Flakes	120	0	0	2
Kellogg's Corn Flakes	110	0	1	2
Post Toasties	107	0	1	2
Health Valley F/F Honey Clusters & Flakes	93	0	3	3
Kellogg's Product 19	110	0	1	3
Kellogg's Rice Krispies	110	0	1	3
Kellogg's Special K	110	0	1	3
General Mills Total Corn Flakes	110	0	1	3
General Mills Corn Chex	110	0	1	3
General Mills Kix	120	1	1	3
General Mills Wheat Chex	108	1	3	3
Health Valley F/F Almond Granola O's	129	0	3	3
Health Valley F/F Apple Cinnamon Granola O's	129	0	3	3
Post Grape Nuts	103	1	3	4
Health Valley F/F Honey Puffed Corn	104	0	3	4
Kellogg's Crispix	110	0	1	4
General Mills Wheaties	110	1	3	4
Health Valley F/F Crisp Brown Rice	89	0	1	4
Quaker Oats Oatmeal Squares	118	2	2	5
Healthy Choice Brown Sugar Squares	106	1	3	5
Kellogg's All-Bran	80	1	10	5
General Mills Total Whole Grain	110	1	3	5
Post Grape Nuts Flakes	103	1	3	5
Kellogg's Strawberry Squares	98	1	3	5
Quaker Oats King Vitamin	116	1	1	6
Post Bran Flakes	100	1	5	6
Kellogg's Nutri-Grain Golden Wheat	100	1	4	6
Kellogg's Complete Bran Flakes	100	1	5	6
Kellogg's Common Sense Oat Bran	110	1	4	6

Food Name	Calories	Fat	Fiber	Sugar
General Mills Body Buddies Natural Fruit	120	1	1	6
Post Honey Bunches Of Oats Honey Roasted	120	2	1	6
General Mills Kaboom	120	2	1	6
Kellogg's Blueberry Squares	98	1	3	6
General Mills Multi-Bran Chex	103	1	4	6
Kellogg's Frosted Mini-Wheats	104	1	3	7
Kellogg's Just Right w/Crunchy Nuggets	109	1	2	7
Kellogg's Apple Cinnamon Squares	98	1	3	7
Kellogg's Raisin Squares	98	1	3	7
Quaker Crunch Bran	100	1	6	7
Quaker Original Toasted Oatmeal	116	1	2	7
Nabisco Frosted Shredded Wheat Bite Size	110	1	3	7
Morning Traditions Blueberry Morning	120	2	1	7
Nabisco 100% Bran	83	1	8	7
Kellogg's Frosted Mini-Wheats Bite Size	104	1	3	7
As Compared To				
Sun Country Granola With Almonds	142	5	2	6
Post Honey Bunches Of Oats w/almonds	126	3	1	7
Quaker Honey Nut Toasted Oatmeal	122	3	2	7
Quaker 100% Natural Granola Oats & Honey	138	5	2	8
Kellogg's Just Right Fruit & Nut	115	1	2	8
General Mills Basic 4	109	2	2	8
Post Fruit & Fiber Peaches, Raisins & Almonds	115	2	3	8
Kellogg's Bran Buds	70	1	11	8
Healthy Choice Granola w/Raisins	110	2	2	8
General Mills Oatmeal Crisp Almond	120	3	2	8
Healthy Choice Almond Crunch w/ Raisins	109	1	3	8
Quaker Life Cinnamon Oat	114	1	2	8
Healthy Choice Granola w/o Raisins	116	2	2	9
Kellogg's Apple Raisin Crisp	98	0	2	9
Kellogg's Fruitful Bran	93	1	3	9
General Mills Honey Nut Clusters	115	1	2	9
Kellogg's Low Fat Granola	115	2	2	9
Kellogg's Mueslix Crispy Blend	109	2	2	9
Kellogg's Nutri-Grain Almond Raisin	109	2	2	9
Kellogg's Low Fat Granola w/ Raisins	115	2	2	9
General Mills Raisin Nut Bran	109	2	3	9
Kellogg's Rice Krispies Treats	120	2	0	9
Kellogg's Temptations French Vanilla Almond	120	2	1	9
Sun Country Granola Raisin And Date	130	4	2	9
Post Fruit & Fibre Dates, Raisins & Walnuts	115	2	3	9
Healthy Choice Mueslix				
Raisin & Almond Crunch With Dates	109	2	2	9
Quaker Frosted Flakes	114	0	1	9
Quaker Low Fat 100% Natural Granola w/Raisins	114	2	2	10
Kellogg's Raisin Bran	93	1	4	10
Kellogg's Nutri-Grain Golden Wheat & Raisin	98	1	3	10
Kellogg's Nut & Honey Crunch	120	2	1	10

Food Name	Calories	Fat	Fiber	Sugar
Kellogg's Cracklin' Oat Bran	126	4	3	10
Kellogg's Frosted Bran	100	0	3	10
Kellogg's Temptations Honey Roasted Pecan	120	3	1	10
Quaker Oats Cap'n Crunch's Peanut Butter	123	3	1	10
General Mills Cinnamon Toast Crunch	130	4	1	10
Post Raisin Bran	97	1	4	10
General Mills Total Raisin Bran	98	1	3	10
General Mills Crispy Wheaties 'N Raisins	104	1	2	11
General Mills Oatmeal Crisp Raisin	115	1	2	11
General Mills Honey Nut Cheerios	120	2	2	11
Kellogg's Apple Cinnamon Rice Krispies	110	0	1	11
Kellogg's Nut & Honey Crunch O's	120	2	2	11
Post Honeycomb	114	1	1	11
Quaker Cap'n Crunch Deep Sea Crunch	126	2	1	12
Kellogg's Frosted Krispies	110	0	0	12
Kellogg's Double Dip Crunch	110	0	0	12
Kellogg's Pop-Tarts Crunch Frosted Brown Sugar Cinnamon	120	1	1	12
General Mills Cookie Crisp	120	1	0	12
Post Alpha Bits	122	1	1	12
Quaker Oh!S Honey Graham	123	2	1	12
Quaker Oats Cap'n Crunch Crunchberries w/Wildberry Colors	115	2	1	13
Quaker Cap'n Crunch Xmas Crunch	115	2	1	13
Kellogg's Frosted Flakes	120	0	0	13
Kellogg's Cocoa Krispies	120	1	0	13
Kellogg's Corn Pops	110	0	1	13
General Mills Lucky Charms	120	1	1	13
General Mills Trix	120	2	0	13
General Mills Apple Cinnamon Cheerios	120	2	1	13
Post Fruity Pebbles	122	1	0	13
Quaker Oats Cap'n Crunch	122	2	1	13
Quaker Quisp Sweet Crunch	122	2	1	13
Post Cocoa Pebbles	124	1	0	13
Kellogg's Apple Jacks	110	0	1	14
Kellogg's Froot Loops	120	1	1	14
General Mills Cocoa Puffs	120	1	0	14
General Mills Boo Berry	120	1	0	14
General Mills Count Chocula	120	1	0	14
General Mills Frankenberry	120	1	0	14
Kellogg's Fruity Marshmallow Krispies	110	0	0	14
Kellogg's Cinnamon Mini Buns	120	1	1	14
Kellogg's Pop-Tarts Crunch Frosted Strawberry	120	1	0	14
Post Marshmallow Alpha Bits	124	1	0	14
Quaker Cocoa Blasts	118	1	1	15
Kellogg's Smacks	110	1	1	16
Post Golden Crisp	122	0	0	17

Tip

As a rule less sugar is better than more. Also, check the fat content, as a few, such as granola, are higher than others. Important to watch serving sizes as bowls can hold 2–3 oz. instead of one.

Chicken Nuggets

Food Name	Calories	Fat	S.Fat	Sodium
Better Choice				
Tyson Chicken Breast Tenderloin	250	7	1.5	330
As Compared To				
McDonald's Chicken McNuggets, 4 Piece	190	11	3	340
Wendy's Chicken Nuggets, 5 Piece	230	16	3	470
McDonald's Chicken McNuggets, 6 Piece	290	17	4	510
Banquet Chicken Nuggets Meal	430	23	8	650
Swanson Chicken Nuggets Dinner	590	25	7	990
McDonald's Chicken McNuggets, 9 Piece	430	26	5	770

Tip

Chicken Nuggets are high in fat; a burger may be the better choice. The problem is the amount of breading as compared to the amount of meat. Consider serving boneless, skinless chicken breast, or use my recipe for chicken nuggets, or serve a frozen, breaded chicken breast or tenderloin.

Crackers

Serving size is about 1 oz., less than 3 grams of fat per serving for the better choices.

Food Name	Calories	Fat	Fiber	Sodium
Better Choice				
Ry Krisp Original	120	0	8	150
Wasa Whole Grain Crisps	103	0	2	17
Health Valley F/F Amaranth Graham	104	0	3	31
Health Valley F/F Whole Wheat Cheese Flavor	107	0	4	171
Keebler Melba Toast, Long	100	0	2	167
Keebler Garlic Melba Rounds	125	0	2	200
Mr. Phipps F/F Original Pretzel Chips	107	0	1	675
Snackwell's F/F Wheat	120	0	2	340
Sunshine Krispy F/F	120	0	1	270
Keebler Zesta F/F Saltines	107	0	1	193
Health Valley F/F No Salt Added Organic Whole Wheat Vegetable	107	0	4	32
Wasa Organic Rye Original Crispbread	94	0	4	188
Manischewitz Tea Matzos, Thin	115	0	0	3
Keebler Selects Low Fat French Vanilla Graham	118	2	1	96
Keebler Selects Low Fat Cinnamon Crisp Graham	118	2	1	204
Wasa Cinnamon Toast Original Crispbread	113	2	2	122
Eden Foods Brown Rice	120	2	2	230
Snackwell's Reduced Fat Classic Golden	129	2	1	300
Pepperidge Farm Pretzel Goldfish	120	3	0	430
Keebler Honey Graham	117	3	3	189
Mr. Phipps Original Pretzel Chips	129	3	1	675
Honey Maid Cinnamon Grahams	131	3	1	197
Triscuit Reduced Fat Wafers	122	3	4	169

Food Name	Calories	Fat	Fiber	Sodium
Premium Soup And Oyster	120	3	1	460
Ralston Animal	134	3	1	83
Sunshine Krispy	129	3	1	386
Premium Original Saltine	129	3	1	386
Harvest Crisps Five Grain	126	3	1	291
Garden Crisps Vegetable	130	3	1	290
As Compared To				
Keebler Wheatables 50% Reduced Fat Original	130	4	1	320
Keebler Munch'ems 55% Reduced Fat Sour Cream & Onion	130	4	0	390
Saltines	130	4	1	391
Keebler Club Partners 33% Reduced Fat Club	131	4	0	375
Sunshine Animal	136	4	0	121
Keebler Wheatables 30% Reduced Fat White Cheddar	130	4	1	330
Keebler Wheatables 30% Reduced Fat French Onion	130	4	1	320
Keebler Munch'ems 55% Reduced Fat Original	130	4	1	450
Wheat Thins Reduced Fat Snack	124	4	2	227
Mr. Phipps Nacho Tortilla Crisps	139	4	3	161
Mr. Phipps Sour Cream 'N Onion Tater Crisps	140	4	1	226
Sunshine Cheez-It Reduced Fat	141	5	0	281
Triscuit Garden Herb Wafers	139	5	3	139
Keebler Munch'ems Original	130	5	1	350
Sunshine Hi-Ho Reduced Fat	140	5	1	280
Keebler Kitchen Rich Grahams	138	6	1	127
Better Cheddars Reduced Fat Baked Snack	140	6	1	350
Keebler Toasteds Compliments Sesame	145	6	1	332
Wheat Thins Snack , Original	145	6	2	176
Wheatsworth Stoned Ground Wheat	150	7	2	253
Keebler Wheatables Original	150	7	1	320
Sunshine Cheez-It White Cheddar	151	7	0	282
Sunshine Hi-Ho Whole Wheat	150	8	1	267
Ritz	150	8	1	253
Ritz Bits Sandwiches With Real Peanut Butter	149	8	1	130
Tid-Bit Baked Cheese Snack	150	8	1	419
Sunshine Hi-Ho	150	9	1	279
Vegetable Thins Snack	155	9	1	300
Chicken In A Biskit Flavored	160	9	1	271
Keebler Town House	164	9	1	281
Ritz Bits Sandwiches Made With Real Cheese	155	10	1	290

Tip:

When it comes to crackers, you can pretty easily convert your usage to the healthier choices. In the first place, you typically use them for snacks rather than as a staple of your daily diet. Secondly, you have quite a variety of "better" crackers from which to choose. So why would you want to keep all those higher fat, lower fiber ones around?

Fish

Serving size is about 3 oz., less than 6 grams of fat for the better choices.

Food Name	Calories	Fat	S.Fat	Sugar
Better Choice				
Mrs. Paul's Baked Fish Sticks	180	3	1	450
Van De Kamp's Crisp & Healthy Fish Sticks	190	3	1	450
Banquet Fish Sticks Meal	132	6	2	373
Gorton's Fish Sticks	176	6	2	377
As Compared To				
Van De Kamp's (Breaded) Fish 'N Fries	173	8	1	168
Van De Kamp's Lightly Breaded Sole Fillet	165	8	2	308
Van De Kamp's Breaded Popcorn Shrimp	205	10	2	463
Gorton's Crunchy Fish Fillets	197	11	3	378
Gorton's Original Seasoning Breaded Shrimp	214	12	2	513
Van De Kamp's Battered Fish Fillet	204	12	2	385
Van De Kamp's Battered Fish Portions	210	13	2	425
Gorton's Potato Crisp Fish Sticks	225	13	3	225
Gorton's Haddock Crispy Batter Fillets	213	13	4	441
Gorton's Baked Scampi Shrimp	233	15	3	382
Gorton's Popcorn Shrimp	243	15	3	560
Gorton's Potato Crisp Fish Fillets	236	15	4	252
Gorton's Crispy Batter Fish Sticks	233	16	4	481
Gorton's Batter Dipped Flounder Fillets	228	17	3	433

Tip
Be careful with adding tartar sauce, which has 17 grams of fat in only 2 tablespoons. Baked fish is better than fried, and the breading can add more than you want of fat and sodium.

Frozen Dessert Bars

Serving size is one bar < 2 grams sat. fat for the better choices.

Food Name	Calories	Fat	S.Fat
Better Choice			
Popsicle	42	0	0
Häagen-Dazs Raspberry and Vanilla Sorbet 'N Yogurt Bars	90	0	0
Luigi's Lemon Italian Ice Squeeze-Up Tube	140	0	0
Weight Watchers Chocolate Mousse Bar	35	1	0
Frozen Pops, Orange Vanilla, Cool 'N Cream	31	1	0
Weight Watchers Chocolate Treat Frozen Dessert	100	1	0
Weight Watchers Orange Vanilla Treat	70	1	1
Sherbet Push Up	91	1	1
Frozen Pops, Chocolate Vanilla	54	2	2
Frozen Pops, Double Chocolate Fudge	55	2	2
Creamsicle	91	2	1
Fudgesicle	104	3	2
Weight Watchers Vanilla Ice Cream Sandwich Bar	160	4	2

Food Name	Calories	Fat	S.Fat
As Compared To			
Baskin-Robbins Cappuccino Blast Ice Cream Bar	120	5	3
Ice Cream Sandwich	144	6	3
Weight Watchers Crispy Pralines 'N Creme Bar	130	7	4
Weight Watchers English Toffee Crunch Bar	120	7	4
Weight Watchers Artic D'lights Frozen Dessert	130	7	4
Weight Watchers Caramel Nut Bar	130	8	4
Baskin Robbins Chocolate Chip Ice Cream, Chillyburger	220	11	7
Baskin Robbins Mint Chip Ice Cream, Chillyburger	220	11	7
Ben & Jerry's Cherry Garcia Yogurt Peace Pop	260	14	9
Baskin-Robbins Tiny Toon Vanilla Ice Cream Bar	210	16	9
Baskin-Robbins Ice Cream Bar, Jamoca Almond Fudge	280	17	9
Ben & Jerry's Vanilla With Heath Coffee Crunch Peace Pop	330	22	14
Ben & Jerry's Vanilla Peace Pop	330	23	16
Häagen-Dazs Vanilla & Milk Chocolate Ice Cream Bar	330	24	14
Ben & Jerry's Chocolate Cookie Dough Peace Pop	420	25	14
Häagen-Dazs Coffee & Almond Crunch Ice Cream Bar	360	26	15
Baskin-Robbins Ice Cream Bar, Peanut Butter Chocolate	340	27	11
Häagen-Dazs Vanilla & Almond Ice Cream Bar	370	27	14
Häagen-Dazs Chocolate & Dark Chocolate Ice Cream Bars	400	27	18
Häagen-Dazs Vanilla & Dark Chocolate Ice Cream Bar	390	27	18

Tip

Ice pops and ice cream bars are a favorite dessert. By providing a bar, a child can finish the entire thing. Portion control is easier. Look how dramatically the fat and saturated fat can add up. Your children will probably enjoy a fudgesicle as much or more than a Häagen-Dazs bar.

Lunchables

Serving size is one Lunchable

Food Name	Calories	Fat	S.Fat	Sugar
Oscar Mayer Low Fat Turkey & Pacific Cooler	360	9	5	42
Oscar Mayer Low Fat Ham & Fruit Punch	330	9	5	34
Oscar Mayer Low Fat Ham & Surfer Cooler	390	11	5	41
Oscar Mayer Extra Cheesy Pizza	300	13	7	3
Oscar Mayer Pepperoni Pizza	310	15	7	3
Oscar Mayer Turkey & Surfer Cooler	430	15	8	46
Oscar Mayer Extra Cheesy Pizza & Fruit Punch	450	15	9	35
Oscar Mayer Pepperoni Pizza & Orange	460	16	8	34
Oscar Mayer Ham & Fruit Punch	440	20	9	40
Oscar Mayer Turkey & Pacific Cooler	450	20	9	40
Oscar Mayer Ham & Swiss	340	20	10	4
Oscar Mayer Turkey & Cheddar	350	20	11	5
Oscar Mayer Deluxe Turkey & Ham	370	21	10	8
Oscar Mayer Ham & Cheddar	360	22	11	5
Oscar Mayer Deluxe Chicken & Turkey	390	23	11	8
Oscar Mayer Bologna & Wild Cherry	530	28	13	46
Oscar Mayer Bologna & American	470	35	17	5

Tip

Avoid at all cost. They are shown here only so you can see how bad these really are. Even the so-called low-fat ones! These have too much fat and sugar. Create your own "lunchable" with zip-locked bags of low-fat deli meat, low-fat crackers or pretzels, water or juice and fruit.

Lunch Meat—Bologna

These values are for a serving size of 2 oz. Generally, in prepackaged meats, each slice is 1 oz. In meats from the deli, the number of ounces per slice will depend on the size and thickness of the slice.

Food Name	Calories	Fat	Sodium
Better Choice			
Oscar Mayer Free Bologna	41	0	568
Healthy Choice:			
Deli-Thin Low-Fat Bologna	60	2	478
Low Fat Beef Bologna	71	2	487
Low Fat Bologna w/Turkey, Pork & Beef	61	2	487
As Compared To			
Louis Rich Turkey Bologna	101	7	548
Lebanon Bologna, Beef, Sliced	120	8	760
Oscar Mayer Light Beef Bologna	122	8	629
Oscar Mayer Light Bologna	122	8	629
Turkey Bologna	113	8	499
Mr. Turkey Turkey Bologna	135	11	754
Pork Bologna	140	11	673
Bologna, Beef And Pork	179	16	579
Beef Bologna	177	16	557
Oscar Mayer Wisconsin Made Ring Bologna	183	16	467
Oscar Mayer Bologna	183	16	588
Oscar Mayer Beef Bologna	183	16	629
Oscar Mayer Garlic Bologna	180	16	582

Tip

Stick with the leanest listed choices since children tend to eat these foods frequently. Add as much as you want of tomatoes, lettuce, or pickles

Lunch Meat—Chicken

These values are for a serving size of 2 oz. Generally, in prepackaged meats, each slice is 1 oz. In meats from the deli, the number of ounces per slice will depend on the size and thickness of the slice.

Food Name	Calories	Fat	Sodium
Better Choice			
Healthy Choice Cold Cuts Oven Roasted Chicken Breast	51	0	487
Healthy Choice Deli-Thin Sliced Oven Roasted Chicken Breast	53	0	494
Hillshire Farm Deli Select Smoked Chicken Breast	50	0	568
Tyson F/F Mesquite Flavored Oven Roasted Chicken Breast	47	0	595

Food Name	Calories	Fat	Sodium
Tyson F/F Hickory Smoked Chicken Breast	47	0	609
Tyson F/F Honey Flavor Chicken Breast	47	0	609
Tyson F/F Oven Roasted Chicken Breast	47	0	622
Tyson F/F Oven Roasted Peppered Chicken Breast	47	0	649
Oscar Mayer Free Oven Roasted Chicken Breast	49	0	710
Mr. Turkey Deli Cut Smoked Chicken	56	0.1	714
Louis Rich Carving Board Classic Baked Chicken Breast	50	0.6	669
Louis Rich Carving Board Grilled Chicken Breast	50	0.6	669
Louis Rich Carving Board Honey Chicken Breast	57	0.6	669
Louis Rich Cold Cuts Oven Roasted Deluxe Chicken Breast	61	1.0	669
Healthy Choice Deli-Thin Smoked Chicken Breast	63	1.6	494
Louis Rich Deli Thin Oven Roasted Brand Chicken Breast	66	1.6	677
Healthy Choice Fresh Trak Oven Roasted Chicken Breast	71	2.0	487
Healthy Choice Cold Cuts Smoked Chicken Breast	61	2.0	487

As Compared To

Louis Rich Cold Cuts Oven Roasted White Chicken	81	5.1	710
Land O' Frost Thin Sliced Smoked Chicken	96	5.6	744

Tip

Almost all chicken is a great low-fat lunch choice.
Be careful about adding regular mayo. Choose mustard instead or light/nonfat mayo to flavor your sandwiches.

Lunch Meat—Ham

These values are for a serving size of 2 oz. Generally, in prepackaged meats, each slice is 1 oz. In meats from the deli, the number of ounces per slice will depend on the size and thickness of the slice.

Food Name	Calories	Fat	Sodium
Better Choice			
Oscar Mayer Free Ham, Baked Cooked	42	0	628
Louis Rich Carving Board Brand Ham Honey Glazed, Thin Carved	66	1	710
Hillshire Farm Deli Select Honey Ham	60	1	598
Healthy Choice Boneless Honey Ham, Water Added	71	2	426
Oscar Mayer Smoked Cooked Ham	54	2	685
Louis Rich Carving Board Brand Ham Honey Glazed	63	2	707
Oscar Mayer, Ham, Lower Sodium	63	2	469
Mr. Turkey Smoked Turkey Ham	66	3	644

As Compared To

Ham, 11% Fat	103	6	748
Oscar Mayer, Ham Chopped	101	6	690
Ham, Chopped, Canned	136	11	775
Ham, Minced, Sliced	149	12	707

Tip

Keep ham a healthy lunch or dinner choice by avoiding regular mayo. Use mustard, horseradish, or nonfat or reduced-fat mayo.

Lunch Meat—Salami

Food Name	Calories	Fat	Sodium
Better Choice			
Louis Rich Turkey Salami	81	5	568
As Compared To			
Mr. Turkey Turkey Cotto Salami	99	7	478
Turkey Salami	111	8	570
Louis Rich Specialties Turkey Salami	122	9	507
Oscar Mayer Beef Cotto Salami	122	9	751
Oscar Mayer Cotto Salami	142	10	568
Beerwurst, Pork, Beer Salami	135	11	704
Oscar Mayer Salami For Beer	136	11	716
Beef Salami, Cooked, Sliced	149	12	668
Beerwurst, Beef, Beer Salami	187	17	584
Oscar Mayer Genoa Salami	210	19	1031
Oscar Mayer Hard Salami	210	19	1073
Pork Salami, Dry, Sliced	231	19	1284
Pork And Beef Salami, Dry	237	20	1056

Tip

Salami is in no way healthy. If your child insists on eating it and nothing else, consider the top two choices. *Remember, you decide what comes into your kitchen.*

Lunch Meat—Turkey

Food Name	Calories	Fat	Sodium
Better Choice			
Louis Rich Cold Cuts Hickory Smoked, Fat Free Breast	51	0	609
Oscar Mayer Smoked, Fat Free Breast	44	0	623
Louis Rich Oven Roasted Breast Of Turkey	51	0	629
Louis Rich Deli Thin Cold Cuts F/F, Oven Roasted Breast	44	0	664
Louis Rich Hickory Smoked Breast Of Turkey Slices	51	0	740
Hillshire Farm Deli Select Smoked	50	1	598
Hillshire Farm Deli Select Oven Roasted	50	1	618
Louis Rich Carving Board, Traditional Carved	50	1	682
Louis Rich Carving Board Hickory Smoked	50	1	682
Healthy Choice Deli, Browned	51	1	365
Louis Rich Specialties Turkey Pastrami	71	2	598
Louis Rich Turkey Pastrami	61	2	649
Mr. Turkey Turkey Pastrami	62	2	596
Mr. Turkey Turkey Ham	66	3	644
As Compared To			
Louis Rich Turkey Salami Cooked	81	5	568
Land O' Frost Thin Sliced Smoked Turkey	88	5	792
Mr. Turkey Turkey Cotto Salami	99	6	478
Louis Rich Turkey Bologna	101	7	548

Food Name	Calories	Fat	Sodium
Turkey Salami	111	7	570
Turkey Bologna	113	8	499
Louis Rich Specialties Turkey Salami	122	9	507
Mr. Turkey Turkey Bologna	135	11	754

Tips

Turkey is a great lean food choice except for turkey/bologna, turkey/salami, or turkey/pastrami. Use mustard instead of mayo or light nonfat mayo to flavor your sandwiches.

Lunch Meat Toppings

Food Name	Amount	Calories	Fat Grams
Mayo, regular	1 tbsp	100	11
Mayo, light	1 tbsp	50	5
Mayo, fat-free	1 tbsp	12	0
American cheese	1 oz	110	9
Catsup	1 tbsp	16	0
Mustard	1 tbsp	20	0
Pickle Relish	1 tbsp	20	0
Sauerkraut	1/2 cup	20	0
BBQ sauce	1 tbsp	25	0
Horseradish	1 tsp	2	0

Macaroni & Cheese

Serving size is about 8 oz. or about 1 cup.

Food Name	Calories	Fat	S.Fat	Sodium
Better Choice				
Annie's Fettuccine w/Cheese and Broccoli Sauce	270	3	2	470
Annie's Bunny Shape Pasta	280	4	2	390
Annie's Shells and Cheddar	280	4	2	390
As Compared To				
Franco-American Macaroni & Cheese	210	7	3	1060
Weight Watchers Macaroni & Cheese Entree	280	7	4	590
Kraft Deluxe Macaroni & Cheese	300	10	6	840
Banquet Macaroni & Cheese Meal	320	11	4	970
Kraft Velveta Shells & Cheese	370	13	9	1050
Macaroni &Cheese, Prepared w/Cheese Sauce	390	16	8	800
Stouffer's Macaroni & Cheese Entree	330	17	6	940

Tip:

Prepare your own macaroni and cheese at home. That way YOU control the amount of butter and cheese, which is where all that fat comes from.

Manicotti

Serving size is 4 ½ oz. About one cup, cooked.
Better choices have < 9grams of fat, < 3 sat. fat, < 30% of calories from fat
Ranked from least to most fat, then saturated fat.

Food Name	Calories	Fat	S.Fat	%Fc
Better Choice				
Weight Watchers Cheese Manicotti Entree	127	3	2	24
Healthy Choice Manicotti w/Three Cheeses Entree	123	4	1	27
As Compared To				
Stouffer's Cheese Manicotti Entree	171	8	4	42
Budget Gourmet Cheese Manicotti				
w/Meat Sauce Entree	189	10	5	47
Bernardi Cheese Manicotti	267	12	7	42
Bernardi Large Cheese Manicotti	256	12	8	42
Celentano Manicotti	400	16	6	36

Tip
For a quick, easy meal, serve one of the "Better Choices" with tomato sauce and a green salad.

Pasta Sauce

Serving size is about 4.5 oz or ½ cup, except for the cream sauce, which is 2 oz. or about ¼ cup. Better choices have <3 grams of fat and <10 grams of sugar.

Food Name	Calories	Fat	S. Fat	Sodium	Sugar
Better Choice					
Healthy Choice					
Super Chunky Mushroom &					
Sweet Pepper Pasta Sauce	45	0	0	390	6
Garlic & Herb Original	50	0	0	390	7
Italian Style Veg. Original	40	0	0	390	7
Super Chunky Veg. Primavera	45	0	0	390	7
Super Chunky Mushroom	40	0	0	390	8
Traditional Original	50	0	0	390	8
Ragu					
Light Chunky Mushroom	50	0	0	390	8
Light Tomato & Herb	50	0	0	390	9
Light Garden Harvest	50	0	0	390	9
Light No Sugar Added	60	2	0	390	5
Five Brothers					
Summer Tomato Basil	60	2	0	470	7
Garden Vegetable Primavera	70	3	0	500	7
As Compared To					
Ragu Gardenstyle					
Super Vegetable Primavera	110	4	1	480	10

Food Name	Calories	Fat	S. Fat	Sodium	Sugar
Chunky Tomato, Garlic & Onion	120	4	1	550	13
Chunky Mushroom & Onion	120	4	1	560	13
Chunky Green & Red Pepper	120	4	1	570	13
Super Mushroom	120	4	1	540	14
Ragu Hearty					
Italian Tomato	120	3	1	580	12
Sauteed Onion & Mushroom	110	4	1	550	14
Parmesan	120	4	1	630	15
Flavored w/Sauteed Beef	130	5	1	580	11
Sauteed Onion & Garlic	130	5	1	530	16
Five Brothers					
Marinara w/Burgundy Wine	80	4	1	480	8
Sauteed Mushroom	90	4	1	460	8
Alfredo w/Mushrooms	80	7	4	490	1
Alfredo	120	11	7	430	1

Tip

Notice that the cream-based sauces (Alfredo) are low in sugar. That's because their tastiness comes from the high concentration of fat! With so many "better" choices to select from, experiment with several *till* you discover your family's favorites.

Pizza

I include pizza because children feel it is a staple of their diet and to deprive them of it would be a crime. You know my philosophy—your kids need to be able to live an enjoyable life, and that means doing what their peers do—like order pizza. However, I'm sure you know by now that the typical pizza is *not* a healthy choice. In general, you can improve on its values a bit if you order *light* on the cheese and ask for some type of vegetable rather than meat. My family enjoys a thin crust with onions, green peppers, and mushrooms, and half the cheese of a standard pizza.

Serving size is about 4 oz., or about the size of *one* slice from a *medium* pizza.
Better choices have less than 9 grams of fat, less than 30% of calories from fat.
Ranked from least to most fat, then saturated fat.

Food Name	Calories	Fat	S.Fat	%Fc
Better Choice				
Round Table Salute Veggie Pizza, Pan Crust	209	6	3	24
Tombstone Light Vegetable Pizza	205	6	2	26
Weight Watchers Deluxe Combo Pizza	229	7	2	26
Round Table Salute Veggie Pizza, Thin Crust	201	7	3	30
Pizza Hut Veggie Lover's Hand Tossed Pizza	234	7	3	26
Round Table Garden Delight Pizza, Pan Crust	226	7	4	28
Tombstone Light Supreme Pizza	219	7	3	30
Weight Watchers Extra Cheese Pizza	268	8	3	28
Weight Watchers Pepperoni Pizza	276	9	3	28
Pizza Hut Hand Tossed Supreme Pizza	270	9	5	30
As Compared To				
Tombstone Deluxe Original 12-in. Pizza	255	12	5	41
Pizza Hut Pan Supreme Pizza	292	13	5	39

Caroline J. Cederquist, M.D.

Food Name	Calories	Fat	S.Fat	%Fc
Celeste Large Deluxe Pizza, Frozen	248	13	4	46
Pizza Hut Pepperoni Lover's Hand-Tossed Pizza	314	13	6	37
Round Table Pepperoni Pizza, Thin Crust	317	15	6	42
Tombstone Pepperoni Original 12-in. Pizza	295	15	7	47
Jeno's Combination Pizza, Crisp 'N Tasty	294	16	4	48
Totino's Pepperoni Party Pizza	294	16	4	50
Pizza Hut Pan Italian Sausage Pizza	319	16	5	46
Pizza Hut Pepperoni Lover's Pan Pizza	338	16	8	44
Tombstone Supreme Thin Crust Pizza	286	17	8	52
Celeste Large Pepperoni Pizza, Frozen	290	17	6	51
Pizza Hut Meat Lover's Pan Pizza	325	17	5	48
Tombstone Pepperoni Thin Crust Pizza	325	20	9	56

Tips
Reduce the fat content of any pizza by removing some of the cheese.
When ordering ask them to "go light on the cheese."
At pizzerias ask them to make pizza without added oil.
Get veggie toppings or stick with cheese only. Avoid any meat toppings.

Popcorn - microwave

Serving size indicated for each brand. Less than 30% of calories from fat, less than 3 grams of fat, less than 1 gram saturated fat.

Food Name	Calories	Fat	S. Fat	%Fc	Sodium
Better Choice					
Jolly Time—America's Best 94% F/F, 3 cups	60	trace	0	0	150
Pop-Secret 94% F/F, 3 cups	60	trace	0	0	120
Orville Smart Pop Microwave Popcorn, 3 cups	45	trace	0	0	72
Healthy Choice Microwave Popcorn, 3 cups	50	1	0	18	165
Newman's Own Light Butter Flavor, 3.5 cups	110	3	1	25	90
As Compared To					
Pop-Secret Light—Butter, 3 cups	70	3	1	39	240
Orville Light Movie Theater Microwave Popcorn, 4.5 cups	110	5	1	37	320
Jolly Time— Butter-Licious, 3 cups	105	6	1	51	120
Jolly Time—White & Buttery, 3 cups	106	6	2	51	210
Jolly Time—Blast O Butter, 3 cups	135	9	3	60	225
Newman's Own Butter, 3.5 cups	170	11	2	58	180
Newman's Own Natural, 3.5 cups	170	11	2	58	180
Orville Ultimate Butter, 4 cups	160	12	3	68	440
Orville Movie Theater Butter Popcorn, 4.5 cups	170	12	3	64	360
Pop Secret Movie Theater Butter Flavor Popcorn, 4 cups	180	13	3	65	300
Orville Movie Theater Microwave Popcorn— Pour Over, 4 cups	170	14	4	74	330

Tips

It is easy to eat the whole bag in one sitting. Divide out popcorn into bowls and let each child and adult have their own serving without needing to compete for more!

Potato Chips

Serving Size: 1 oz. Better choices include < 30% of cals from fat < 3 grams of fat, < 1 gram sat fat, < 220 mg sodium.

Food Name	Calories	Fat	S. Fat	% Fc	Sodium
Better Choice					
Auburn Farms F/F Original	99	0	0	0	138
Auburn Farms F/F Cheddar	99	0	0	0	168
Louise's F/F Original	110	0	0	0	180
Michael Season's French Onion Baked	110	2	0	12	150
Guiltless Gourmet Baked, Lightly Salted	110	2	0	12	180
Baked Lay's	110	2	0	16	180
Utz Baked	110	2	0	16	220
Baked Ruffles	120	3	0	23	200
Baked Ruffles Cheddar & Sour Cream	120	3	1	23	220
As Compared To					
Michael Season's Lightly Salted, 40% Less Fat	130	6	1	42	80
Cape Cod 40% Reduced Fat	130	6	0	42	110
Ruffles Reduced Fat Regular	130	7	1	46	160
Lay's Sour Cream & Onion	150	9	3	54	180
Ruffles KC Masterpiece Mesquite BBQ	150	9	3	54	190
Barbara's Bakery Yogurt & Green Onion	150	9	1	54	240
Pringles	160	10	0	56	160
Ruffles Original	150	10	3	60	180
Lay's Original	150	10	3	60	180
Ruffles French Onion	150	10	3	60	180
Ruffles Cheddar & Sour Cream	160	10	3	56	190
Lay's Deli Style Cheddar	150	10	3	60	190
Lay's KC Masterpiece BBQ	160	10	3	56	200

Tips

Choose baked chips but be careful about portion sizes. Serve in individual bowls rather than from the bag.

Pretzels

Serving Size: 1 oz. Best choices have <30% of cals from fat; < 3 grams of fat; < 1 gram of sat fat; < 200 mg sodium.

Food Name	Calories	Fat	S. Fat	% Fc	Sodium
Better Choice					
Harry's Honey Mustard or Ranch	100	0	0	0	95
Michael Season's Mini Organic, Unsalted	120	1	0	8	30

Food Name	Calories	Fat	S. Fat	% Fc	Sodium
Harry's Everything	110	1	0	8	120
Barbara's Bakery Honeysweet Pretzels	100	1	0	9	135
Barbara's Bakery Mini Pretzels, No Salt Added	100	1	0	13	30
Barbara's Bakery Bavarian Pretzels	100	2	0	14	170
As Compared To					
Rold Gold F/F Tiny Twist Pretzels	100	0	0	0	420
Louise's F/F Sourdough Pretzels	90	0	0	0	470
Mister Salty Mini Pretzels	110	1	0	8	441
Michael Season's Mini Organic, Lightly Salted	120	1	0	8	300
Rold Gold F/F Hard Sour Sough	110	1	0	8	370
Rold Gold Crispy Thin Twist Pretzels	110	1	0	8	420
Mister Salty Dutch Pretzels	120	1	0	8	580
Barbara's Bakery Mini Pretzels	100	1	0	13	290
Keebler Mini Pretzels	120	2	0	11	660
Sargento Mootown Snackers Cheeze & Pretzels	90	3	2	30	320

Tips

Most pretzels are low in fat, but some still have too much sodium to be healthy. Watch portion sizes and serve in bowls rather than from the bag. Read labels carefully to make sure you are buying a "better" choice instead of one high in sodium.

Ravioli

Best choices have less than 4.5 grams of fat, less than 3 grams of saturated fat, less than 30 percent of calories from fat). Ranked from least to most fat, then saturated fat.

Food Name	Calories	Fat	%Fc	S.Fat
Better Choice				
Weight Watchers Smart Ones Florentine Entree	101	1	9	0
Chef Boyardee Cheese in Tomato Sauce w/Beef	114	2	12	1
Healthy Choice Cheese Parmigiana Entree	131	3	17	1
Chef Boyardee Beef in Tomato And Meat Sauce	121	3	20	1
Trio's LowFat Cheese	300	3	9	1
Celentano Great Choice Low Fat Cheese	250	3	11	1
Chef Boyardee Mini Beef in Tomato & Beef Sauce	122	3	23	1
Stouffer's Lean Cuisine Cheese Entree	127	4	26	2
As Compared To				
Franco-American Superior Beef in Meat Sauce	158	5	29	2
Amy's Kitchen Cheese w/Sauce	162	6	32	1
Bernardi Square Cheese	226	6	24	3
Stouffer's Lunch Express Cheese	173	7	35	2
Contadina Light Garden Vegetable	347	7	19	4
Contadina Light Cheese	349	7	19	3
Lucca Beef	286	8	24	2
Bernardi Square Beef	244	8	29	4
Lucca Italian Sausage w/Herbs & Seasonings	301	9	27	2
Bernardi Jumbo Beef (Round)	269	11	38	5
Contadina Cheese	412	18	39	9

Tip

Remember we want to keep fat to less than 30 percent of our daily calories. As with other pasta dishes, choose a nonoily tomato sauce rather than a cream-based sauce and add a green salad.

Serving size is 4 ½ oz. —About one cup, cooked.
Better choices include < 7 grams of fat, < 3 grams saturated fat, < 30% of calories from fat.

Tortellini

Ranked from least to most fat, then saturated fat.

Food Name	Calories	Fat	%Fc	S.Fat
Better Choice				
Gina Italian Village Meat Tortellini	340	4	11	2
Romance Tortellini Florentine	240	4	15	2
Bernardi Cheese Tortellini	260	6	21	3
Contadina Mushroom And Cheese Tortellini	360	7	18	2
As Compared To				
Bernardi Tortellini Variety Pack	256	8	28	4
Bernardi Spinach Tortellini w/Cheese	280	8	26	5
Trio's Cheese Tortellini	370	9	22	3
Contadina Three Cheese Tortellini	380	9	21	5
Contadina Cheese Tortellini	393	9	21	4
Digiorno Mozzarella Garlic Tortellini	390	10	23	6
Contadina Chicken & Vegetable Tortellini	400	11	24	3
Digiorno Three Cheese Tortellini	390	11	25	5

Tip

Instead of serving with a cream-based sauce, choose a tomato sauce without any oil. Add a mixed green salad for a tasty and healthy meal.

This concludes our listings of better, healthier choices as compared to those that you probably should scratch off your shopping list. Remember—after a few weeks of eating the healthier varieties, your family's tastes will adapt to the new foods and you won't miss the ones you formerly ate. Well, you won't miss them enough to want to return to those unhealthy habits.

Appendix Four

Meanings of Key Words on Food Labels

The government has defined what food labels mean when they use certain words. Following is a list of key words and their meanings, courtesy of the American Heart Association. All definitions are "per serving."

Calorie Free: Fewer than 5 calories

Light (Lite): 1/3 fewer calories or no more than 1/2 the fat of the higher-calorie, higher-fat version; or no more than 1/2 the sodium of the higher-sodium version

Fat-Free: Less than 0.5 gram of fat

Low Fat: 3 grams of fat (or less)

Reduced or Less Fat: At least 25% less fat per serving than the higher-fat version

Lean: Less than 10 grams of fat, 4 grams of saturated fat and 95 milligrams of cholesterol.

Extra Lean: Less than 5 grams of fat, 2 grams of saturated fat, and 95 milligrams of cholesterol.

Low in Saturated Fat: 1 gram saturated fat (or less) per serving and not more than 15 % of calories from saturated fatty acids

Cholesterol Free: Less than 2 milligrams of cholesterol and 2 grams (or less) of saturated fat.

Low Cholesterol: 20 milligrams of cholesterol (or less) and 2 grams of saturated fat (or less).

Reduced Cholesterol: At least 25% less cholesterol than the higher-cholesterol version, and 2 grams (or less) of saturated fat

Sodium Free: Less than 5 milligrams of sodium per serving, and no sodium chloride (NaCl) in ingredients

Very Low Sodium: 35 milligrams of sodium (or less)

Low Sodium: 140 milligrams of sodium (or less)

Reduced or Less Sodium: At least 25% less sodium than the higher-sodium version

Sugar Free: Less than 0.5 gram of sugar

High Fiber: 5 grams of fiber (or more)

Good Source of Fiber: 2.5 to 4.9 grams of fiber

Don't try to memorize these. Just note that the key words follow the same pattern for each nutrient, i.e., "free" bears the least amount; "very low" and "low" have a little more; "reduced" or "less" always refers to a food with 25 percent less of that nutrient than the standard version of that food.

Complementing Protein Foods

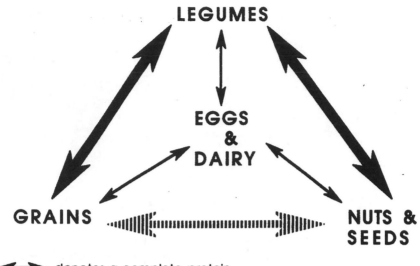

→ denotes a complete protein

··ıll:···}ıₙ·· denotes an incomplete protein-
low in the same amino acid

Here are some examples of meals you might plan to use several times a week, as these complementing proteins deliver complete protein without meat.

1) cereal + *skim* milk

2) pasta (macaroni/spaghetti) + cheese

3) sandwich made with whole grain bread + cheese or eggs

4) beans + rice or other whole grain

5) pasta + beans

6) barley + pinto bean soup

7) peanut butter (natural) sandwich on whole grain bread + milk

8) baked beans + whole grain bun

9) bean soup + whole grain bread

Suggested Serving Sizes

Food Group	Servings	1-3 yrs	3-6 yrs	6-12 yrs	12+ & Adults
Bread, Cereal, Grains	7 - 11 per day	1/2 slice or 1/4 c	1/2 slice or 1/3 c	1 slice or 1/2 c	1 slice or 1/2 c
Vegetables	3 - 5 per day	1/4 c	1/3 c	1/2 c	1/2 c
Fruits	2 - 4 per day	1/4 c	1/3 c	1/2 c	1/2 c
Milk & Milk Products	2 - 3 per day	1/2-3/4c	3/4-1c	1 cup	1 cup
Meat & Meat Alternates	2 - 3 per day	1 oz or 1/4 c	11/2 oz or 1/3 c	2 oz or 1/2 c	2-3 oz or 1/2 c

Food Choices for Good Health
Breads and Cereals

Often:
Whole grains or enriched breads
English muffin
Bagels
Tortillas, flour or corn
Rice, white and brown
Pita bread
Cooked cereals
Ready-to-eat UNsugared cereals
Spaghetti
Macaroni
Noodles
Matzo
Breadsticks
Grits, boiled
Fat-free or low-fat crackers
Pretzels
Graham crackers

Sometimes:
Pancakes
Waffles

RARELY:
Croissants
Doughnuts
Sweet rolls
Granola
Ready-to-eat *sugared* cereals
Cheese crackers
Pastries
Corn chips
Tortilla chips
Granola bars
Fried grits
Snack crackers

Fruits and Vegetables

Often:
All fresh fruits and vegetables
Canned vegetables
Fruits canned in juice
Plain frozen vegetables
Vegetable juices
Soups, including cream soups made with
    nonfat milk
Frozen fruit-juice bars

Sometimes:
Fruits canned in light syrup
Vegetables frozen w/butter
    or other sauce
Pickles, olives
RARELY:
French fries
Fruits canned in heavy syrup
Hash browns
Canned cream soups
Frozen fruit-*flavored* bars

Meat, Poultry, Fish, Eggs, Beans and Nuts

Often;
Well-trimmed, lean cuts of beef, pork
    veal and lamb
Chicken and turkey without skin

Fish and shellfish, *not fried*
Peas (split, chick, black-eyed)
Beans
Extra lean ground beef
Tuna canned in water
Refried beans made without lard
Light or reduced-fat meat products

Sometimes:
Eggs
Peanut butter
Peanuts, pistachios, cashews,
    macadamia nuts, walnuts,
    almonds, pecans, beechnuts
    Brazil nuts, filberts
Pumpkin and sunflower seeds
Tofu

RARELY:
Bacon, sausage, frankfurters
Bologna, Salami
Deep fried chicken
Deep fried fish
Tuna canned in oil
Ground beef with 30% fat
Refried beans made with lard
Ham hocks and salt pork

Milk and Dairy Products

Often:
Nonfat milk
Reduced-fat milk
Cottage cheese, reduced fat
Chocolate milk, reduced fat
Buttermilk made from skim or low-fat milk
Nonfat or low-fat dry milk
Low-fat cheeses such as ricotta,
    mozzarella
Cream cheese, nonfat

Sometimes:
Cheese made with whole milk,
    such as cheddar, jack, or Swiss
Cottage cheese
Frozen yogurt
Sherbet
Ice cream, reduced fat, low-fat or light
Pudding made with nonfat milk
Flan or custard made with skim milk
Cream cheese, light, or reduced fat

RARELY:
Whole milk
Ice cream
Sour cream
Cream cheese
Half and half
Chocolate milk
Heavy/whipping cream

Sweets, Fats, Snack Foods

Often:
Unbuttered popcorn
Fresh fruits and vegetables
Bagels, small (not chocolate chip)
Frozen fruit-juice bars
Low-fat or nonfat yogurt
Fat-free salad dressings
Ready-to-eat UNsugared cereals

Sometimes:
Margarine, reduced fat
Salad dressings, reduced fat
Mayonnaise, reduced fat
Diet soft drinks
Cookies
Butter, reduced fat
Pretzels & baked chips

Rarely:
Butter
Margarine
Vegetable oil
Salad dressing
Candy
Chocolate
Sugar
Honey
Jelly, jam, marmalade, preserves
Soft drinks
Fruit-flavored drinks
Rich sauces
Gravies
Potato or corn chips
Granola

Remember portion control!

Want to Calculate Your BMI?

* Here is the formula used to calculate the Body Mass Index:

$$\frac{\text{weight (in pounds)}}{\text{height (in inches)}^2} \times 703 = BMI$$

[handwritten: $\frac{158}{65.5 \times 65.5}$]

or, using the metric system:

$$\frac{\text{weight (in kilos)}}{\text{height (in meters)}^2} = BMI$$

[handwritten: 65.5]

How Do Your Parents Measure Up?

The World Health Organization has developed three categories of adult obesity.

* BMI 25 to 29.9 = Grade 1 (moderate overweight) *[handwritten: 25.88]*
* BMI 30 to 39.9 = Grade 2 (severe overweight)
* BMI over 40   = Grade 3 (massive/morbid obesity)

Using the formula, we can compute that an adult whose height is 5 feet 7 inches and weight is 150 pounds would have a *body mass index* of 23. A glance at the three WHO categories tells you that this person would not be considered over-weight. On the other hand, a 5-foot 10-inch person weighing 210 pounds with a BMI of 30 would be considered severely overweight. A person's health risk from obesity increases as the BMI increases.

Resources

* Persons wishing to obtain a referral to a bariatrician—a licensed physician who has received special training in bariatric medicine—in their state of residence may call 303-779-4833 or send an e-mail to **bariatric@asbp.org**. Be sure to include your complete mailing address. Additional information about obesity and the ASBP can be found by logging onto **http://www.asbp.org**.

* Other resources:

http://www.drcederquist.com

American Obesity Association**,** Morgan Downey, Executive Director and CEO; 1250 24th St. NW, Suite 300, Washington, DC 20037; phone: 202-776-7711; fax: 202-776-7712—obesity advocacy, research, community action.

Appendix Five

Recipes from the Cederquist Kitchen

From time to time in the first six chapters of this book, I indicated that you would find several healthy recipes that my family has tried, liked, and continued to keep as part of our meal planning and enjoyment. I have divided these recipes into **SNACKS, BREAKFAST**, **LUNCH**, and **MAIN MEALS**. Some snacks are suitable for taking along—to school, to the playground, or wherever— and I'll point those out. Others are best eaten at home, perhaps after school when kids are typically dehydrated and famished. You can rest assured that my kids, ages eight and six as this book goes to press, not only eat these foods without protest, they actually request them. And that's saying a lot, considering that one of them loves all the junky foods I have advised against throughout this book.

Snacks

Pretzels

Spread nonfat cream cheese on the top of a large pretzel and especially in the holes. Refrigerate. Kids can grab this when they come home from school. It satisfies that need for a crunch plus a little protein.

Stuffed Celery, Garnished Apples, and Cucumber

Cut celery into 2-inch lengths, cut apples into wedges and core, slice cucumbers.

For stuffing you can use nonfat cream cheese or natural peanut butter. And to make things interesting you can press whole almonds on the top, or sprinkle the top with raisins, chopped dates, apricots or other dried fruits, sunflower seeds, or other nuts. Without the cream cheese (which should be kept cold), these snacks can go into the kids' backpacks for munching in mid-morning between classes or anytime.

Humptee Dumptee

This is the name our family uses for hard-boiled eggs to which we add a bit of salt-free seasoning (paprika or Mrs. Dash). Believe it or not, I've discovered through working with patients that not everyone knows how to boil an egg, so here's the recipe. Forgive me if you feel insulted, but I just want to be sure!

1) Place eggs in a pan and cover with enough cold water to go an inch above the tops of the eggs.
2) Bring water to boil.
3) Reduce heat and simmer for 12 minutes.
4) When time is up, run under cold water. Peel and run under cold water again if you are going to use them immediately. Unpeeled, boiled eggs placed in the fridge will keep fresh for close to a week.
5) Cut eggs in half and sprinkle with seasoning.

Green Eggs and Ham

Our family tribute to Dr. Seuss!

2 hard-boiled eggs
1 1/2 Tbs. nonfat cream cheese
1 1/2 Tbs. shredded reduced-fat cheddar cheese
1 1/2 Tbs. lean ham, finely chopped
salt and pepper to taste

Cut eggs in half and discard yolks. In a small bowl, mix together all remaining ingredients. For fun, you could add green food coloring or parsley. Divide evenly and press into the yolk cavity of the egg white. Enjoy right away or wrap with foil and refrigerate for later.

Fruit Salad

Serving varies

You can add just about any type of fruit you like (fresh or frozen). Any combination will be scrumptious, but here are some ideas.

1) bananas, strawberries and pineapples or
2) blueberries, raspberries and blackberries or
3) apples, oranges and bananas
plain fat-free yogurt, cinnamon, honey

Combine all fruit in a medium bowl. Mix in yogurt, cinnamon, and honey to taste.

Variations:
1) For a light breakfast, serve in the center of a cantaloupe half.
2) To balance with a protein, add either almonds or pecans. But if you are packing this for lunch, remember to pack the nuts separately and add later when ready to eat.

Stuffed Apple Volcanoes

Apples
Chunky natural peanut butter

1) Wash apples and slice off the top.
2) Core the apple to remove seeds.
3) Stuff with chunky natural peanut butter.
4) Put top of apple back on and wrap in foil if it will be eaten later.

Variation:
Add raisins and low-fat granola. You can either sprinkle mixture over the top of the apple or add to the peanut butter.

Fruit Banana Split

Serves 4

4 bananas
2 cups low-fat cottage cheese (1% preferred)
Large can of fruit cocktail, packed in natural juices only

Cut each banana into four pieces and put in bowl. Add 1/2 cup cottage cheese on top of bananas. Cover with fruit cocktail.

Cooked Fruit

Apples, pears or bananas
cinnamon or cinnamon-sugar

Cut apples or pears into quarters and core. Cut banana in half lengthwise.

Sprinkle fruit with cinnamon or cinnamon-sugar. In a nonstick pan (no oil) over medium-low heat, slowly cook fruit until soft. Serve hot. Although great for a snack, it does require a responsible person to do the chores at the stove. As an alternative, microwave until fruit is soft, 1.5 to 3 minutes. This can also be used as a dessert. This also tastes great served with nonfat vanilla yogurt on top.

Frozen Fruit

Frozen fruit makes a wonderful treat and has a completely different appeal than fresh fruit. Try frozen blueberries, pineapple chunks, strawberries, and grapes; buy them frozen or freeze them yourselves. They are delicious and a real cool treat.

Fruit and Vegetable Dips

Okay, I promised you some low-fat dips to use with veggies in order to get your kids into the habit of eating veggies. Here are a couple that work extremely well.

Orange Dipping Sauce

1/2 cup nonfat ricotta cheese or plain nonfat yogurt
2 Tbs. orange-juice concentrate
1/2 tsp. vanilla extract

Place all ingredients in a small bowl and mix until smooth.

Raspberry Dipping Sauce

1/4 cup nonfat cream cheese
1/4 cup nonfat vanilla yogurt
2 Tbs. raspberries, fresh or frozen

Place all ingredients in a small bowl and mix until smooth.

Variation:
Replace raspberries with strawberries.

Ravioli Trail Mix

You can buy trail mix at the store, but you need to be very careful to check what's in it—like preservatives, sugar. Also, it can be pricey. Try making your own; it is fun and easy! It is great for snacking or for food on the run.

Mix any of the following ingredients or try your favorite. Sunflower seeds; raisins; whole almonds; carob chips; chunks of coconut; pumpkin seeds; Chex cereal. Just mix together and keep in a tightly covered container or place small servings into plastic bags so the kids (and grown-ups too) can grab them from the pantry as needed.

Homemade Potato Chips

1–2 lbs. potatoes
1-2 Tbs. olive oil
coarse salt, if desired

Preheat oven to 400 degrees. Wash potatoes and slice paper thin. Place all ingredients into a large plastic bag and shake well. Spread out on a baking sheet and bake crisp, about 15 minutes.

Homemade Salsa

Remember to adjust seasonings—especially the jalapeños—to your kids' tastes.

1 28 oz. can diced tomatoes, drained
1 4.5 oz. can green chilies, chopped
2 cloves garlic, minced
1 tsp. sugar
2 tsp. apple cider vinegar
1/2 tsp. salt
1/2 tsp. cumin
3/4 cup onion, finely chopped
1 Tbs. lime juice
jalapeño pepper, fresh or bottled, to taste (optional)
1/4 cup fresh cilantro, chopped

Mix all ingredients in a large bowl. Refrigerate for an hour or more. Serve with baked chips.

Variation:
Try adding 1 15-oz. can of black beans, rinsed and drained. It's a nice change in flavor and is a great source of protein and fiber.

Breakfast

Cornmeal-Blueberry Pancakes

Makes 8 large pancakes

1 cup all-purpose flour
1/2 cup yellow cornmeal
1 to 2 Tbs. honey, syrup, or sugar
2 tsp. double-acting baking powder
1 egg plus 1 egg white
2 tbs. vegetable oil
1 cup nonfat buttermilk
1 cup fresh or frozen unsweetened blueberries

1) Sift the flour, cornmeal, sugar, and baking powder together.
2) In a mixing bowl, whisk together egg, egg white, oil, and nonfat buttermilk.
3) Add the dry ingredients to the egg mixture and stir gently just until the flour is blended in; do not overmix.
4) Stir in blueberries.
5) Heat a large nonstick griddle over medium heat until a few drops of water sprinkled onto the surface skip about and evaporate almost instantly.
6) Spoon about 1/3 cup of batter into skillet so it makes a pancake about 4 inches across.
7) Cook first side until bubbles begin to form and the underside is browned; turn the pancake over and cook the other side until brown.

Variation:
Replace blueberries with thinly sliced apples, peaches, or bananas.

Blueberry-Orange Syrup

Makes 1 1/2 cup

This syrup is delicious whether it is made with fresh, frozen, or canned fruit. If you are using canned fruit, please remember to use the kind packed in juice rather than in syrup.

1 1/2 cup unsweetend blueberries
1/4 cup orange-juice concentrate

1) Put the blueberries into a small saucepan and stir in the orange-juice concentrate.
2) Bring the mixture to a simmer over low heat, stirring frequently until heated through. Serve warm.

Variation:
1) Replace blueberries with thinly sliced apples, peaches, or bananas. Use your imagination to create flavors your kids will love.
2) Omit the orange-juice and simmer only the fruit until it becomes a compote.

Lunch

Creamy Tuna Salad

Serves 4

1 6-oz. can water-packed tuna, drained
3/4 cup nonfat ricotta cheese
2 1/2 Tbs. reduced-fat or nonfat mayonnaise
1 Tbs. sweet pickle relish
2 Tbs. finely chopped onion
1/4 cup finely chopped green or red pepper
1/4 cup finely chopped celery
salt and pepper to taste

In a bowl, combine all ingredients, mixing well. Serve on whole wheat bread with your child's favorite toppings—fresh tomatoes, pickles, alfalfa sprouts, etc.

Variation:
Substitute onion, peppers, and celery with:
1/2 cup finely chopped apple
2 Tbs. sunflower seeds
1 Tbs. raisins
or
1 medium carrot, grated
1/3 cup raisins

Note: Tuna salad tastes better if you can chill several hours to blend flavors.

Egg Salad

Serves 6

8 hard-boiled eggs
1/2 cup finely chopped purple onion
1/2 cup nonfat ricotta cheese
2 Tbs. reduced-calorie or fat-free mayonnaise
2 Tbs. Dijon-style mustard
salt and fresh ground pepper, to taste

1) Peel the eggs and chop them in a medium airtight container.
2) Combine all remaining ingredients.
3) Serve with either pita bread or whole wheat bread with your child's favorite toppings—fresh tomatoes, pickles, alfalfa sprouts, etc.

Grilled Ricotta and Jam Sandwiches

Serves 4

8 slices whole-wheat bread
4 tsp. butter
4 Tbs. strawberry or raspberry jam
1 1/3 cup nonfat ricotta cheese

Spread 1/2 teaspoon or less of the butter on one side of each slice of bread. Place buttered side down on a clean work surface. Top four of the bread slices with 1 tablespoon jam and 1/3 cup ricotta cheese. Cover each sandwich with the remaining slices of bread, buttered side up. Place the sandwiches in a large nonstick skillet or on a griddle if you have one over low heat and grill until nicely browned. Serve with your favorite fruit.

Grilled Cheese and Ham Sandwiches

Serves 4

8 slices whole-wheat bread
4 tsp. butter
8 slices reduced-fat or nonfat cheese
4 slices of Canadian bacon (in Canada, known as peameal bacon—go figure!) or low-fat ham

Spread 1/2 teaspoon or less of the butter on one side of each slice of bread. Place buttered side down on a clean work surface. Top four of the bread slices with a slice of cheese, a slice of ham, and another slice of cheese. Cover each sandwich with the remaining slices of bread, buttered side up. Place the sandwiches in a large nonstick skillet over low heat and grill until nicely browned and the cheese is melted. Serve with your favorite fruit.

Variation:
Add a slice of pineapple or tomato to the sandwich.

Baked Potato Skins

Serves 8

Ingredients:
4 medium potatoes
1/2 cup grated fat-free cheddar cheese
3 Tbs. very lean, cooked bacon bits
1/4 cup minced green onion
Freshly ground black pepper and salt, to taste

Preheat the oven to 375 degrees. Scrub potatoes and pierce each all over with the tines of a fork. Place them on a baking sheet and bake until the skin is very crisp, about 1 1/2 hours. Cut potatoes in half lengthwise. Remove the insides of the potatoes and save for another use, leaving a 1/4-inch shell. Cut potato halves lengthwise. Spray potato shells with butter-flavored spray.

Sprinkle evenly with cheese, bacon bits, and green onion and return to oven for 3 minutes longer to melt cheese. Sprinkle with salt and pepper and serve immediately.

Sweet Potato Fries

2 lbs. sweet potatoes or yams
1–2 Tbs. rosemary, chopped
1–2 Tbs. olive oil
coarse salt, if desired

Preheat oven to 375 degrees. Wash sweet potatoes and cut into sticks or wedges. Place all ingredients into a large plastic bag and shake well. Spread out on a baking sheet and bake until browned and tender, about 30 minutes. This makes a nice lunch or can be served as a side dish with a main meal entree.

It's A Wrap

Here's a clever way to get children to eat their vegetables: Give them wrap sandwiches. These need not be reserved for lunch—they can make a great choice for dinner, too. What's more, you can pack in a serving or more of vegetables, not to mention grain and protein. Variations are endless, limited only to your child's imagination. Here are a few suggestions to get you started.

* **Turkey Roll-up.** Spread a whole-grain tortilla with honey mustard and top it with lean deli turkey, low-fat cheese, and shredded carrots. Roll up tightly.

* **Philly Cheese Steak.** Layer lean roast beef, red and green bell-pepper strips, and shredded reduced-fat cheddar cheese on a whole-grain tortilla. Microwave for 30 seconds or until cheese melts, then roll up tightly.

* **Chicken Melt**. Layer warm chunks of chicken, nonfat sour cream, shredded reduced-fat Monterey Jack cheese, chopped tomatoes, and raw spinach on a whole-grain tortilla. Then roll up tightly.

* **Southwestern Wrap.** Layer lean deli turkey, strips of red bell pepper and avocado, bean sprouts, and low-fat Swiss cheese on a whole-grain tortilla. Then—let's see if you've been paying attention—what do you do now? Yep, roll up tightly.

* **Soft Taco.** Spread a whole-grain tortilla with salsa and nonfat sour cream. Top with lean deli roast beef (or lean cooked ground beef, if available), chopped tomatoes, shredded lettuce, shredded reduced-fat Monterey Jack cheese, and taco sauce. Then roll up tightly.

* **Creamy Tuna Melt**. Prepare Creamy Tuna Salad above. Spread over whole-grain tortilla and top with shredded carrots and shredded reduced-fat Monterey Jack. Microwave for 30 seconds or until cheese melts, then roll up tightly.

* **Pizza Wrap**. Spread a whole-grain tortilla with your favorite tomato/pizza sauce. Top with your favorite toppings (turkey pepperoni is okay but vegetables are better) and reduced-fat mozzarella cheese. Microwave for 30 seconds or until cheese melts if you want it hot, or serve cold. Then roll up tightly.

Main Meal Entrees

Pasta with Broccoli and White Beans

1 lb. pasta, cooked (your kids' favorite shape)
1 lb. broccoli, steamed and chopped
1 red bell pepper, cut into strips
4 cloves garlic, minced
1/2 cup reduced sodium, nonfat chicken broth
1 can (15 oz.) white beans, rinsed and drained
salt and pepper, to taste
3 Tbs. chopped fresh basil or 1 1/2 tsp. dried basil
Parmesan cheese
fresh parsley, chopped (optional)

Prepare pasta according to package directions. Steam broccoli. In a large saucepan coated with nonstick spray, over medium heat, add garlic and red pepper. Sauté until tender. Add broth, beans, basil, salt and pepper and bring to a simmer. Heat thoroughly. Combine pasta, broccoli, and bean mixture in a larger bowl and mix well. Top with 1 tablespoon of Parmesan cheese and parsley and serve immediately.

Variation:
You can easily make this dish into a healthy low-fat Pasta Primavera. Just cut back on the amount of broccoli to 2 cups and add 2 cups mushrooms, 2 cups zucchini, 2 cups tomatoes, and 1/2 cup peas. Or add whatever vegetables you have on hand or that your child would eat.

Beef (or Turkey) Chili Nachos

Serves 6

Our Turkey Chili Nachos make for a great main meal. Quick to prepare, the recipe uses 99% fat-free ground turkey. You can replace the turkey with a low-fat ground beef, like *Maverick Beef*.

1 Tbs. olive oil
1 lbs. 99% fat-free ground turkey or low-fat ground beef, like *Maverick Beef*
1 medium onion, chopped
1 clove garlic, minced
1 tsp. dried oregano
½ tsp. chili powder
½ tsp. cumin
salt and pepper to taste
1 14-oz. can black beans, drained
1 cup tomato salsa
corn tortilla chips, preferably baked chips
1/2 cup red pepper, diced
1/2 cup green pepper, diced
jalapeño peppers, minced, to taste
½ cup black olives, optional
1 cup low-fat Monterey Jack cheese, shredded
2 Tbs. fresh cilantro, chopped
guacamole
nonfat sour cream

Heat oil in large skillet over medium-high heat. Stir in turkey, breaking it up with a spoon; cook until no longer pink. Remove. Stir in onion, garlic, oregano, chili powder, cumin, salt, and pepper; cook until onion is soft. Return the cooked turkey, stir in the black beans and salsa; simmer until heated through. Place corn tortillas onto large baking sheet, spoon turkey chili over top. Sprinkle with peppers and olives, if desired. Sprinkle with cheese. Bake at 425 degrees for about 5 minutes or until cheese melts. Top with fresh cilantro and serve with guacamole and sour cream.

Easy Nachos

Serves 2 to 4

16 to 20 plain tortilla chips, baked
1 cup low-fat Monterey Jack cheese, shredded
chopped olives (optional)
sliced green onion (optional)
salsa
nonfat sour cream

Preheat oven to 400 degrees. Spread tortilla chips in a single layer in a baking pan or cookie sheet. Sprinkle cheese over chips. Add olives and green onion. Bake for 2 to 3 minutes or until cheese melts. Serve with salsa and nonfat sour cream.

Chicken Nuggets

Here's the recipe I promised you when the list of prepared nuggets showed how UNhealthy they are!

Serves 4 to 6

1 egg
2 Tbs. milk
1 cup Italian bread crumbs
1 lb. boneless/skinless chicken breast, cut into 1 or 1- 1/2-inch bite-sized pieces
cooking spray

Preheat oven to 400 degrees. Whisk eggs and milk together in a small bowl; set aside. Place bread crumbs in a gallon-sized, zip-top bag. Dip each chicken piece in the egg and milk mixture, then let the kids help by shaking the pieces in the crumb bag. Place each coated nugget on a cookie sheet coated with cooking spray. Bake for 15 minutes or until done. Serve with your favorite low-fat dipping sauce.

Variation:
You can add different seasonings to the bread crumb mixture. Try Mrs. Dash salt-free seasoning, a lemon-pepper season, or for something spicy, try Chef Paul Prudhommes's Poultry Magic. You can also replace the Italian bread crumbs with cornflakes.

My Mother-in-law's Meatballs

1 lb. low-fat ground beef, like *Maverick Beef*
1/4 cup Parmesan cheese
1/2 cup Italian bread crumbs
1 clove garlic, minced
2 Tbs. parsley
1 egg
1/2 tsp. salt
1/2 tsp. black pepper

Preheat oven to 350 degrees. Let your kids mix all ingredients together in a large bowl—disposable gloves or plastic bags are helpful for this—and shape into balls about the size of a golf ball. Place each on a cookie sheet coated with cooking spray. Bake until done, about 15 minutes. Cover with your favorite tomato sauce and serve with pasta.

Macaroni and Cheese

Remember how I said that instead of using prepackaged meals, you could use your own recipe and control the fat content? Well, here's mine.

1 1/2 cup skim milk
4 Tbs. all-purpose flour
1/2 tsp. dry mustard
1/2 tsp. paprika
pinch, cayenne pepper
salt and black pepper to taste
1/2 cup reduced-fat cheddar cheese, shredded
1/4 cup reduced-fat Swiss cheese, shredded
1/2 cup nonfat sour cream
4 cups cooked macaroni
1/4 cup Italian bread crumbs

Preheat oven to 350 degrees. In a large saucepan, combine the milk, flour, mustard, paprika, salt, and peppers until smooth. Cook over medium heat until mixture is bubbly and thickened, about 8 minutes, stirring frequently. Stir in all cheeses. Continue to cook until cheeses are completely melted.

Combine cheese sauce with cooked macaroni. Transfer to a large casserole dish that has been coated with nonstick spray. Sprinkle Italian bread crumbs over macaroni. Bake until hot, about 20 to 25 minutes.

Pasta with Cheese and Ham

Serves 4 to 6

16 oz. pasta, cooked (Use your kids' favorite—shells, spirals, penne)
1 egg plus 1 egg white
1 cup skim milk
3/4 cup grated Parmesan or your favorite reduced-fat cheese
salt and pepper to taste
1/2 cup lean ham, sliced into short, narrow strips
1/2 cup peas (optional)

Mix eggs, milk, cheese, salt, and pepper in a small bowl. In a large nonstick pan over medium heat, lightly sauté the ham until thoroughly warm; remove and set aside. Lower heat and coat pan with nonstick cooking spray. Add the egg and cheese mixture. Cook until edges begin to set, about 30 seconds. Add the cooked pasta, ham, and peas, and raise heat to medium. Stirring constantly, cook until mixture is hot and eggs have thickened, about 3 to 5 minutes. Serve hot.

Tuna Casserole

3 cups cooked macaroni
2 6-oz. cans tuna fish, water packed
1 10.75-oz. can 98% fat-free cream of mushroom soup
1 cup frozen peas, thawed (optional)
3/4 cup onions, chopped and sautéed (optional)
Worcestershire sauce
salt and pepper
1/4 cup parsley, chopped
Italian bread crumbs

Preheat oven to 400 degrees. Drain tuna. Place in a large casserole dish and separate it with a fork. Add soup, peas, and onions, and season with Worcestershire sauce, salt, pepper, and parsley. Combine cooked macaroni and mix. Sprinkle Italian bread crumbs over macaroni. Bake until top is brown, about 15 minutes.

Marinades for Chicken

Instead of buying from the grocery, you can make your own. That lets you control the ingredients, as well as the cost!

Honey-Mustard Marinade

1/3 cup honey
2 Tbs. Dijon mustard
1 clove garlic, minced
1 Tbs. cider vinegar
1 Tbs. soy sauce

Mix well. Marinate chicken 4 to 12 hours, refrigerated. Baste with the marinade during cooking.

Teriyaki Marinade

1/4 cup soy sauce
1/3 cup orange juice
2 Tbs. olive oil
1 Tbs. brown sugar
2 cloves garlic, minced
1 tsp. grated fresh ginger

Mix well. Marinate chicken 4 to 12 hours, refrigerated. Baste with the marinade during cooking.

Fish Sticks—Homemade

This is getting to be a familiar refrain, but it's still true. You can quickly and easily prepare some of your kids' favorites at home instead of buying one of the high-fat varieties. They are still yummy!

1 egg
2 Tbs. milk
1 cup Italian bread crumbs
1/2 tsp. onion powder
dash garlic powder
salt and pepper to taste
1 lb. fish filets (snapper, cod, flounder, etc. cut into sticks)
cooking spray

Preheat oven to 400 degrees. Whisk egg and milk together in a small bowl; set aside. Combine bread crumbs, onion powder, garlic powder, salt, and pepper. Dip each fish stick in the egg and milk mixture, then roll in seasoned bread crumbs. Place on a cookie sheet coated with cooking spray. Bake for 10–15 minutes, turning once. Serve with your favorite low-fat dipping sauce.

Variation:

You can add different seasonings to the bread crumb mixture. Try Mrs. Dash salt-free seasoning, a lemon-pepper season, or for something spicy, try Chef Paul Prudhommes's Seafood Magic. You can also replace the Italian bread crumbs with cornflakes.

Soups

You can serve soups alone for lunch or as part of a main meal. Here are some nice, easy recipes.

Egg Drop Soup with Rice

Serves 4

4 cups reduced-sodium chicken broth
1 cup cooked rice
1 egg and 1 egg white
lemon juice and pepper, to taste

In a medium-sized saucepan, add chicken broth and rice. Bring to a full boil. Stirring the broth constantly with a circular motion, slowly pour in the eggs. Taste the soup for seasoning. Add a little lemon juice or pepper if desired. Serve hot.

Cream of Broccoli Soup

2 heads broccoli (about 2 pounds), finely chopped, tough stem ends trimmed away
1 large onion, chopped
2 leeks, well rinsed and thinly sliced
1 Tbs. olive oil
1 potato, scrubbed and cut into chunks
1 rib celery, chopped
1 carrot, chopped
2 cups water
2 cups skim milk
1/4 tsp. nutmeg
1 tsp. salt
pepper to taste

Sauté onion and leeks in oil over medium heat for 3 to 5 minutes. Add carrots, celery, broccoli, potatoes, and water; simmer until the vegetables are quite tender. Stir in the milk and seasonings. Heat thoroughly and serve immediately.

Corn Chowder

2 cups onions, chopped
2 Tbs. olive oil
2 Tbs. all-purpose flour
2 1/2 cups low-sodium chicken broth
2 large potatoes, peeled and cut into 1/4 inch dice
3 cups corn, frozen or fresh
2 cups skim milk
salt and pepper, to taste
1 large red bell pepper, chopped (optional)
fresh cilantro, for garnish (optional)

In a large soup pot over medium-low heat, sauté onion in oil until white, about 5 minutes. Add flour and cook, stirring another 5 minutes. Add chicken broth and potatoes. Continue cooking until the potatoes are just tender, about 15 minutes. Add corn, skim milk, salt, and pepper. Heat thoroughly. Add the bell pepper and cook an additional 5 minutes. Remove from heat and serve immediately, garnished with cilantro.

Variation:
Add 1/2 to 1 cup diced lean ham while sautéing onions.

Red and White Bean Chicken Chili

Do your kids like their chili spicy? If not, adjust seasonings accordingly.

1 1/2 cup onion, chopped
1 cup celery, chopped
1 cup carrot, chopped
1 cup green bell pepper, chopped
1–3 cloves garlic, to taste, minced
1– 3 Tbs. bottled jalapeño peppers, to taste, minced
1 lb. cooked chicken breast, shredded
1 28-oz. can diced tomatoes, undrained
1 can (14 1/2 oz.) low-sodium, fat-free chicken broth
1 1/2 Tbs. chili powder
2 tsp. ground cumin
1 tsp. dried oregano
1/4 tsp. cayenne pepper (optional)
1 Tbs. unsweetened cocoa
1 can (19 oz.) red kidney beans, drained and rinsed
1 can (19 oz.) white kidney beans, drained and rinsed
shredded reduced-fat cheddar cheese

In a large saucepan coated with nonstick spray add 1/2 cup onion, chopped celery, carrot, green bell pepper, garlic, and jalapeño peppers. Cook over medium-low heat until tender, about 10 minutes. Add remaining ingredients except beans and bring to a boil. Cover, reduce heat, and simmer for 20 minutes. Add beans and heat thoroughly. Remove from heat and serve immediately with a little cheese sprinkled on top each bowl.

Lentil Soup

2 cloves garlic, minced
1 1/2 cup carrots, chopped
2 cups onions, chopped
1 Tbs. olive oil
2 cups lentils, rinsed and drained
6 cups water, or low-sodium, fat-free vegetable or chicken broth
2 tsp. ground coriander
2 tsp. ground cumin
salt and pepper, to taste
1 bag (10 oz.) fresh spinach, prewashed and coarsely chopped

In a large saucepan, heat oil over medium heat. Add garlic, carrots, and onions. Cook until tender, about 5 minutes, stirring often. Add lentils, broth, coriander, cumin, salt, and pepper. Bring mixture to a boil. Reduce heat and simmer until lentils are very soft, about 20 minutes, stirring occasionally. If necessary, add more water to get soup to desired consistency. Stir in spinach, adjust seasoning if needed. Cover and simmer for 5 more minutes or until spinach is tender. Remove from heat and serve immediately.

Once you begin to incorporate these healthier recipes into your at-home meals, I'm sure you'll find ways to vary the ingredients to satisfy the tastes your family most enjoys. It's fun to experiment and discover new dishes. Just remember to use nonfat sprays instead of oil, low-fat meats and cheeses, plenty of no-calorie seasonings, and lots of veggies. Happy and healthy dining!

End Notes

Chapter One References:

1. National Health and Nutrition Examination Survey (NHANES) III, 1988-1994, as quoted in the American Society of Bariatric Physicians (ASBP) June 1999 Talking Paper.
2. *Ibid*.
3. Kennedy, Mark, "Obesity a top threat in the 21st century," *The Windsor Star*, August 26, 2000, pp.1-2.
4. *Pediatric Alert*, March 27, 1997, as noted in the June 1999 Talking Paper of ASBP.
5. "What Is Obesity?" ASBP Talking Paper, June 1999.
6. "New Pediatric/Adolescent Growth Charts Provide Tool to Ward Off Future Weight Problems," *The Bariatrician*, September 2000.
7. Kennedy, p. 2.
8. Charts downloaded from Web site: www.cdc.gov/growthcharts; U.S. Department of Health & Human Services, Centers for Disease Control & Prevention, National Center for Health Statistics, Division of Data Services, Hyattsville, Maryland, 20782-2003.
9. Stunkard, A.J., Sorenson, T., et.al., "An Adoption Study of Human Obesity," *New England Journal of Medicine*, April 1986, pp. 193–198.
10. Griffiths, M., Payne, P.R., "Energy Expenditure in Small Children of Obese and Non-obese Parents," *Nature*, 1976; 260 (5553): 698–700.
11. Griffiths, M., Rivers, J.P., Payne, P.R., "Energy Intake in Children at High and Low Risk of Obesity," *Human Nutrition, Clinical Nutrition*, 1987; 41 (6): 425–430.
12. Patterson, M.L., Stern, S., Crawford, P.B., et.al., "Sociodemographic Factors of Obesity in Preadolescent Black and White Girls," NHLBI's Growth and Health Study, National Medical Association, 1997; 89: 594-600.
13. "The Relation of Overweight to Cardiovascular Risk Factors Among Children and Adolescents: The Bogalusa Heart Study," *Pediatrics*, June 1999, 1175–1182.

Chapter Two References:

1. Alphin, Franca B., MPH, RD, LDN, "Improved Eating Habits for Lifelong Change," lecture delivered at Duke University Diet and Fitness Center program *Setting New Standards in Weight Management*, Durham, North Carolina, July 17, 1999.
2. "Food Consumption, Prices, and Expenditures, 1970-97," Economic Research Service, USDA, from the ERS Web site updated September 18, 2000.

Chapter Three References:

[1]   Liebman, Bonnie, "The Changing American Diet," *Nutrition Action Healthletter*, April 1999, pp. 8-9.
[2]   Wyshak, G., "Teenaged Girls, Carbonated Beverage Consumption, and Bone Fractures," *Archives of Pediatric Adolescent Medicine,* June 2000; 154(6): 610-613.
[3]   Rask-Nissila, Jokinen, et.al., "Neurological Development of 5-year-old Children Receiving a Low-Saturated Fat, Low-Cholesterol Diet Since Infancy," *Journal of the American Medical Association,* August 23, 2000, Vol 284, No 8, p 993-1000.
[4]   Wyshak.
[5]   Ludwig, Majzoub, et.al., "High Glycemic Index Foods, Overeating, and Obesity," *Pediatrics*, March 1999, 1-6.

Chapter Four References:

[1]   Klesges, Shelton, Klesges, "Effects of Television on Metabolic Rate: Potential Implications for Childhood Obesity," *Pediatrics*, February 1993, 281-286.
[2]   Anderson, Crespo, et.al., "Relationship of Physical Activity and Television Watching With Body Weight and Level of Fatness Among Children," *Journal of the American Medical Association*, March 25, 1998, 937-941.
[3]   Gotmaker, S.L., Dietz, W.H. and Cheung, L.W.Y., "Inactivity, Diet and the Fattening of America," *Journal of the American Dietetic Association*, 1990, pp. 1247-1252, 1255.
[4]   Klesges, p. 284.

Chapter Six References:

[1]   Levick, Keith, Ph.D., "Eating Disorders in Adolescence," *The Bariatrician*, Spring 1998, pp.12-14.
[2]   Creighton, Judy, "Encourage Positive Body Image for Kids," The *Windsor Star*, August 30, 2000, p. B5.

Index